PHOTOGRAPHING MEDICINE

Recent Titles in
Contributions in Medical Studies

PHOTOGRAPHING MEDICINE

Images and Power in Britain and America since 1840

Daniel M. Fox *and* Christopher Lawrence

Contributions in Medical Studies, Number 21

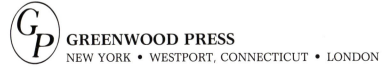

GREENWOOD PRESS
NEW YORK • WESTPORT, CONNECTICUT • LONDON

Library of Congress Cataloging-in-Publication Data

Fox, Daniel M.
  Photographing medicine.

  (Contributions in medical studies, ISSN 0886-8220 ;
no. 21)
  Includes index.
  1. Medicine—Great Britain—History. 2. Medicine—
Great Britain—History—Pictorial works. 3. Medicine—
United States—History. 4. Medicine—United States—
History—Pictorial works. 5. Photography, Medical—
Great Britain—History. 6. Photography, Medical—
United States—History. I. Lawrence, Christopher J.,
1947-   . II. Title. III. Series. [DNLM:
1. History of Medicine, 19th Cent.—Great Britain—
pictorial works. 2. History of Medicine, 19th Cent.—
United States—pictorial works. 3. History of
Medicine, 20th Cent.—Great Britain—pictorial works.
4. History of Medicine, 20th Cent.—United States—
pictorial works. 5. Photography—history—Great
Britain—pictorial works. 6. Photography—history—
United States—pictorial works. W1 CO778NHE no.21 /
WZ 17 F791p]
R486.F69 1988   610'.941   87-25088
ISBN 0-313-23719-0 (lib. bdg. : alk.paper)

British Library Cataloguing in Publication Data is available.

Library of Congress Catalog Card Number: 87-25088
ISBN: 0-313-23719-0
ISSN: 0886-8220

First published in 1988

Greenwood Press, Inc.
88 Post Road West, Westport, Connecticut 06881

Printed in the United States of America

10 9 8 7 6 5 4 3 2 1

CONTENTS

ACKNOWLEDGMENTS

Many people assisted us in the preparation of this book. Most of the American photographs were collected under a grant from the National Endowment for the Humanities for a project conducted by Daniel M. Fox, Martin Pernick, Guenter Risse and Judith Walzer Leavitt with the assistance of Rima Apple and James S. Terry. Antonia Ineson began the collection of the British photographs with Christopher Lawrence. Ghislaine Lawrence, Lynn Szygenda and William Schupbach helped to find other pictures. We also thank the many others who called our attention to photographs or sent them to us.

A number of colleagues helped us to formulate the ideas in the book and to improve the manuscript. Steven Shapin discussed many of the ideas in the text with Christopher Lawrence. Daniel Fox benefited from conversations with Martin Pernick. John Burnham, Martin Pernick and Roy Porter read the manuscript and made helpful suggestions.

Producing a book of this kind requires an unusual amount of support. J. Howard Oaks cheerfully absorbed many of the costs on behalf of the Health Sciences Center of the State University of New York at Stony Brook. Many of the British costs were met by the Wellcome Institute for the History of Medicine. Katherine Stephani word processed the earliest drafts. Rosamond Kelly was a valued coordinator of our work. Sally Wood performed efficiently the difficult task of preparing the final version of the manuscript.

PHOTOGRAPHING
MEDICINE

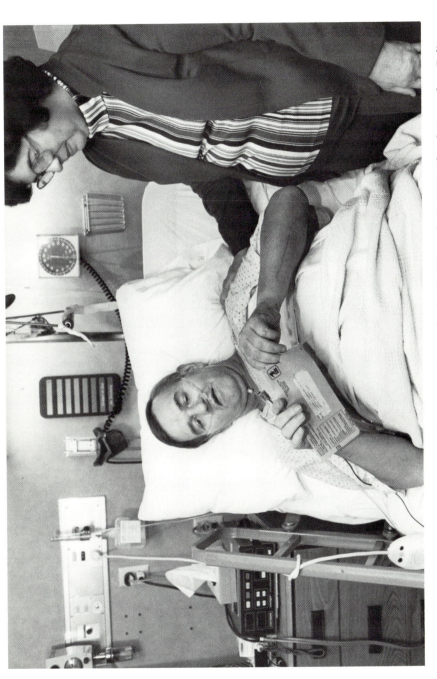

Fig. 0.1 William Schroeder after receiving a heart implant in Louisville, Kentucky in 1984. The photographer, Pulitzer Prize winner William Strode, took the picture for Humana Audubon Hospital (William Strode: Black Star).

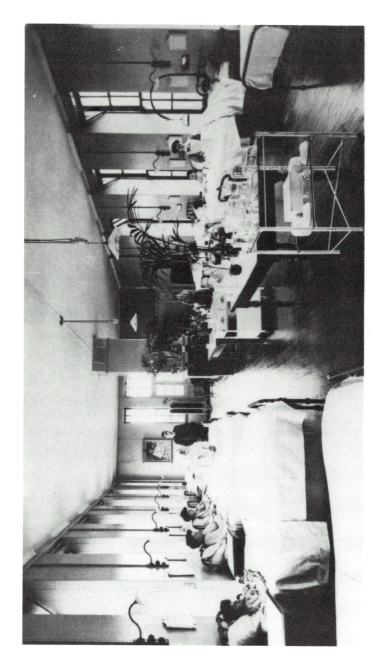

Fig. 0.2 Postcard of a surgical ward at St. John's and St. Elizabeth's Hospital, London, c. 1909. The postcard reads "Dearest Kathleen, what do you think of these nice little white beds? & is it not a pretty room?" (Wellcome Institute Library, London).

PROLOGUE

Consider these two pictures. The first will be familiar to most readers. The other will seem unremarkable to anyone who has looked at old photographs. The first photograph (Fig. 0.1) appeared in newspapers in the United States and abroad in 1984, often on the front page. There are a number of clues in this photograph which seem to identify it as a picture about medicine taken since the Second World War: the technology, the clothing, hair styles, the official envelope, for example. There is, however, rather more to our recognition of it as a contemporary photograph. The way the picture is taken seems modern: the camera angle, the lighting, the people's expressions, the ratio of the space filled by people to the amount of background. When we learn that the man in this picture was the recipient of an artificial heart we can make even more sense of the photograph. It is a picture about medical care, technology, science and skill, but it is also about individuals. It is a human story about a woman and her husband. With little prompting, we can all make up a story about this picture. It is a story about how medicine offers the possibility of a future to this couple. We could also make up other stories about the photograph, for example, about his fortitude and her bravery. Even without any information, we would all probably make up stories like this because, throughout our lives, we have been taught how to read these messages in photographs of this sort.

The second photograph (Fig. 0.2) was taken in a British surgical ward around the turn of the century. We know that, like the previous photograph, it was intended for public display, since the hospital issued it as a picture postcard. As in the first picture, there are clues, such as the design of the light fittings, which seem to settle its date. But, again, like the first picture, the camera angle, the lighting, the way the people occupy the space, identify it as a photograph taken at a particular time. Just as the first photograph seems automatically to tell the modern observer something, so, too, the ordinary viewer in 1910 could have made up a number of stories about medicine and hospital patients on the basis of this picture. The stories would probably have been about the efficiency of voluntary hospitals in providing up-to-date and orderly surgical treatment for the poor. Like the modern viewer, the observer at the turn of the century would have learned how to read particular meanings in such photographs.

Each of these photographs resembles many others taken around the same time. The first picture looks like most of the photographs of medicine that have appeared in the press since the 1940s—close-up representations of patients. The second picture is a typical medical photograph from the years around the turn of the century. The photograph is unmistakably about an institution rather than individuals.

In this book we discuss many more pictures like these. We try to clarify how the composition of medical photographs permits their relatively accurate dating. In addition, we will show how the historical context in which these compositions were viewed constrained viewers to make up a particular set of stories about the photographs. Finally, we will suggest that photographs have a history, and that pictures like these have been among the means by which medical power has been legitimated and extended.

CHAPTER I

IMAGES AS HISTORY

This book is a history of the photographic representation of medicine in Britain and the United States since the 1840s. It began when we both set out, independently, to collect photographs as an extension of our work in other areas of the history of medicine in these two countries. Each of us soon discovered, however, that photographs pose profound problems of historical interpretation. A photograph or series of them can be the basis of many plausible stories. Historians who purport to tell of the past simply by displaying photographs are actually relying on their readers to impute meaning to the pictures from their knowledge of the past and their system of values. When they are not directed, readers will always provide a text, a plausible story, in private. For photographs to be used as the basis of an historical study they must be accompanied by an interpretation, just like any other historical source. This interpretation must be grounded in a coherent theory that explains why people at a particular time represented themselves in particular ways.

This book is a study of pictures as documents: of the meanings contemporaries would have given to them and the uses to which they were put. We have tried to read the photographs in conjunction with other primary sources and the best historical accounts of the recent past. The result is a book of more than 250 photographs, which we think are representative of the thousands we have seen, and a text which is intended to tell readers what we think people in the past tried to say with these pictures and how various audiences would have read and used them. We have no doubt that sometimes we are wrong in our interpretation of how people understood a picture, but we believe that, in the main, we have recovered some of the meanings given to these photographs by those who saw them.

The central subject of the book is the way that orthodox medicine has used photography to represent itself. Our purpose is to describe how the camera, because of its putative capacity to copy reality, was one of the means by which orthodox medicine made its professional image into a public one. Most pictures of medicine have been produced in situations where the power was in the hands of medical orthodoxy: doctors, hospital governors, or the women at the top of nursing hierarchies. Their perceptions of medicine prevailed when photographs were taken, selected, or rejected. Orthodox medicine, of course, has never been a monolithic body, and another book could be written about the use of different sorts of imagery by different medical interests. Although we explore some of these differences here, those between specialists and general practitioners for instance, it is not our primary aim.

The number of photographs of medicine, and the variety of situations in which they were taken, have increased enormously since the announcement of Daguerre's discovery in 1839. This numerical increase can, using other sources, be interpreted as evidence of the growing power and prestige of the medical profession and of the increasing presence of medicine in people's lives. In addition to this simple increase, however, photographs have also represented medicine differently at different times. The historical challenge is to show how these changing representations were related to changes in medical power.

Photographs, then, should enable historians to do more than tell a familiar story using a different sort of document. Photographs can be used to arrive at new understandings of the past. From them we can learn about people's ways of seeing—how images were created and used, how they carried messages about what to value and how to behave. Photographs are, to adapt a definition from Raymond Williams, a *"signifying system* through which . . . a social order is communicated, reproduced, experienced and explored."[1]

Historians have had an ambivalent relationship with photographs. Because modern history remains a literary discipline with roots in philology and philosophy, a work which uses photographs is often dismissed as a "coffee table book," an entertainment for people who like old pictures. Historians, however, have frequently used photographs either to supplement accounts based on written sources or as "illustrations" to "prove" a factual point made from textual analysis. Photographs, paradoxically, are considered too obvious to merit the historian's close attention yet also are used as windows through which the past can be viewed with great accuracy.

In recent years, this "historical-windows" concept has been challenged by a number of scholars who have become interested in studying photographs as problematic historical documents. Two areas of enquiry have emerged. On the one hand there are detailed, empirical studies which interpret photographs using methods adapted from the history of art. Most of this work has been done by critics and historians of photography and literature. On the other hand sociologists of knowledge have produced theoretical and empirical studies that analyse photographs as extremely complex representations made by the use of conventions.[2]

Photographs are the hard case for the study of how reality is constructed by societies because, for most of their history, they have been considered as the "norm of truthfulness," that is, as the standard against which other accounts are to be judged.[3] For this reason, this study is limited to photographs alone. Had we analysed the representation of medicine in painting or drawing, for instance, we would be open to the charge that we were dealing with individual interpretations which could therefore be biased in contrast to the depictions of photography. Thus we decided to limit the book to the historical study of those representations of medicine generally considered to be unambiguously "truthful." For this reason, we also avoided photographs which people would have regarded as "fakes": for example, some of the pictures used in drug advertising. However, such a distinction is difficult to make since many photographs used in advertising would have been read as depicting actual events. (See Fig. 5.55 for an obvious example, but there are many others throughout the book).

Since the 1840s almost everyone has taken it for granted that photographs, unlike hand-made pictures, invariably froze or copied an instant of reality. In our previous metaphor, they have been looked at as windows which offered a privileged view of past events. Although, initially, a few intellectuals were concerned about "photographic distortion" eventually nearly everyone agreed that the camera copied the world. Emile Zola, a keen amateur photographer, declared in 1901, for instance, that, "you cannot claim to have really seen something until you have photographed it."[4]

Although the advocates of photography credited it with the power to copy the world exactly, in fact the technique merely made it easier and cheaper to record and duplicate the sort of images which for centuries artists had made by hand. The forerunners of the modern camera were devices which were invented during the Renaissance. These first cameras were machines built to make pictures using the newly described rules of perspective. According to Renaissance theories of perception, pictures made by using such rules looked like objects seen with the naked eye. In the first cameras, light entered an enclosed box through a lens and an image was projected onto a screen. A permanent copy of this image was made by drawing. In the early nineteenth century, inventors replaced drawing with chemical means of copying and preserving the image. The mechanical and photochemical bases of the process were, in turn, used as evidence for the verisimilitude of photographic prints. To all observers, the camera appeared to provide images which, whether they were used as scientific evidence, public records, or private remembrances all "looked like" the object which had been photographed and, therefore, could not be misunderstood. A typical reviewer in a nineteenth-century medical journal, for example, pointed to "the value of the art of photography to medical and scientific men as a means of recording the experience of the eye."[5]

The modern camera was invented in order to produce and fix two dimensional representations of the world. Later, other technologies were devised for duplicating the images, thus making possible their wide distribution. The representational language which the photograph uses has had a long historical genesis in western art and is learned anew by all of us. It is for historical reasons that we describe the patterns of light, shade and color on a photographic print as "looking like" what we see. The photochemical process involved in making a print, however, only guarantees a constant relation between image and object, not that the image is a *copy* of the photographed object. In order to make a picture that we *call* a copy, photography must be carried out such that it satisfies many socially constructed criteria.

To meet these criteria photographers and their subjects use a number of conventions. Proper use of these conventions permit photographer and subject to compose the image required in a particular instance. The conventions which have been used in making the photograph can be seen in the print. The conventions relating to the proper use of light, for example, require familiarity with the technology of the camera. To begin with, the photographer must allow light to enter the camera from a conventionally defined angle. Similarly, the amount of light allowed through the lens and the time for which the plate is exposed are varied, according to convention, in different circumstances. Sometimes by accident or design these conventions are not properly observed and the result may be condemned as over-exposed or blurred. In depicting speed or eroticism, however, "blurring" is sometimes considered desirable, and the use of the appropriate conventions produces it.

The particular conventions which are used when people are photographed depend on the social roles which are to be represented. For example, families assemble with the children looking bored, surgeons wear white coats or, more recently, green suits, models take off or display their clothes, and generals put on their medals. A "good" or "truthful" picture is one which successfully uses the appropriate conventions to translate into the language of the photograph people's perceptions of themselves and their world. Most of the pictures that remain as historical documents are of course "good" pictures, that is, they are the ones which people kept because they were made by using the appropriate conventions. The "poor" print or the "objectionable" photograph can therefore be an important source for understanding how people see the world.

Photographic conventions are immensely adaptable. For example, the conventions for representing the family were sometimes transferred to other contexts. In Figure 3.10 the staff of a ward and perhaps a patient at the Boston City Hospital in the 1870s were represented as a family. By contrast in Figure 3.13 the people in a British ward scene of the 1890s were not represented in this way.

Changes in the photographic conventions which are being used at a particular time should signal to the historian changes in self-perception by those involved in producing the photograph, and, therefore, changes in the messages which were meant to be read in the picture. A change in a photographic convention, however, should not be interpreted as an indication of a corresponding change in social relations. In the early days of photography, for instance, men were usually represented seated and women standing, a convention often used in British hospital pictures, for example in Figure 3.54. Today the reverse is usually the case, women sit and men stand, but no one would want to suggest there has been a complete reversal of the sexual division of labor and authority in medicine.

Many of the conventions employed in making early medical photographs were those which were used in paintings and drawings to produce portraits and domestic scenes. Photographers drew on these conventions, using them in all areas of medicine in order to represent, for instance, sick people, treatment, and doctors, individually or in groups. At first, therefore, nearly all medical pictures were little different from those depicting everyday affairs. In early clinical photographs for example, a patient's social class could usually be deduced from his or her dress, demeanor, or surroundings (Figs. 1.1, 1.2). By the 1890s, however, photographers began to employ distinctive conventions to differentiate clinical photographs, both from other depictions of medicine and from any other sort of picture. Because many of the basic conventions used in current clinical photography were produced at the turn of the century, clinical photographs from that time resemble much more those taken today than they do those produced in the 1850s and 1860s. We discuss this point more fully in the next chapter.

In the twentieth century, publicly available photographs of medicine have, increasingly, represented it as a distinctive activity. The conventions employed in making these pictures have gradually been changed during this century. They have been changed in order to communicate new messages about medicine. Examining the changes in the conventions used to construct these images, therefore, permits a description of how people have been variously educated into ways of seeing medicine in Britain and the United States.

Besides studying the conventions employed in making photographs, it is crucial to know the context in which pictures were used. Photographs of medicine have been used to publicize, to advertise, to instruct, to celebrate, to create a personal or institutional record and occasionally to criticize or to amuse. The same photograph might have been employed in all these contexts. Conventions and context of use are, of course, not unrelated. The intended use of a photograph determines the conventions which are adopted to present particular subjects. When we do not know their context of use, pictures become ambiguous documents. It is disconcerting to acknowledge that many of the photographs we have examined were not accompanied by any documentary evidence about their employment. In a way this situation resembles that of the historian confronted by an anonymous fragment of text which might be open to numerous interpretations. However, we think it possible to surmount this difficulty and, in many instances, make generalizations about how photographs were read.

Photographs, of course, can be used as a rather different sort of documentary source, just like any other historical text. They can be used by historians of dress or artifacts to establish details about life in the past. In many ways they are very useful for this purpose. Often a great deal can be gleaned more quickly from a photograph than from a printed text. But they are not a *privileged* source; like every other historical document they have been made by a social process. The appearance of a particular artifact in a photograph still behooves the historian to treat the document with the same circumspection that would be appropriate for any other source. Our concern here, however, is not with this use of photographs but rather with understanding the meanings that contemporaries gave them.

We chose the photographs that appear in this book, whether conventional or unconventional, because they are useful for understanding the history of the commonest images of medicine. This choice led us to emphasize the medical profession and its penumbral world. What we leave out is not unimportant to the history of medicine: it is just not central to its visual history. For instance, in our research we have found relatively few images of practitioners of such non-orthodox activities as faith healing, chiropractic and patent medicine sales. The context in which these pictures circulated almost always remains obscure, and their paucity suggests that they were marginal to the making of the predominant medical image. Nor have we included photographs of orthodox medical practices—cupping or leeching for instance—which became *visually* obsolete fairly early in the period we describe. Cupping and leeching were used in medicine until the 1930s, but representing these practices was not, judging from the absence of photographs, considered important. By contrast, for example, the representation of the therapeutic use of electricity was extremely common in the 1920s. Finally, we have excluded photographs of events such as political campaigns or exposures of inadequate housing and working conditions because they were not used to construct a distinctive visual image of medical care. We have, however, included a few photographs of civic activities that pertain to public health. These photographs, we suggest, directed public attention to matters that were increasingly perceived as within the mandate of medicine.

Colleagues have suggested that we divide photographs of medicine into those that were destined for private and those intended for public use. However, except in a few interesting cases, we can discern no difference in the conventions used in those medical photographs that we know were meant for private circulation and those that we know were meant for public display. We have classified photographs of medicine into two broad categories defined by how much we know about the conventions employed to make them, the context of their use and, where it exists, written evidence about them. In one category are the pictures about which we know a great deal, for example, those taken in the late 1930s by photojournalists working for *Life* in the United States and *Picture Post* in Britain. We can learn who took them, when, why, how they were used and how the audience was expected to read them. Moreover, the composition of these photographs is particularly distinctive because these magazines self-consciously took the lead in creating and refining a new style; the visual language of photojournalism.

In the other category are the majority of pictures in this book. These are the sort of photographs that are usually found in abundance in hospital and public archives or private commemorative albums. We have no documentary evidence concerning the individual use of most of them. When these photographs were made within a few years of each other, however, they almost always resembled one another because their makers employed the current conventions. Because we do know how a number of these pictures were used, and because the others have similar origins, we believe it is legitimate to infer that similar photographs were used and read in similar ways.

Within this category there are also pictures of which we have unusual versions in which the familiar conventions were not employed. The significance of these pictures is that they demonstrate that there were other possible ways of representing the medical world. For example, in 1920, a photographer in New York City took at least two photographs of a group of philanthropists visiting a ward for sick children (Figs. 4.45, 4.46). One of these photographs employs the conventions for depicting people as a family. The second picture is quite unlike any other picture of people in American hospitals that we have seen. It does resemble other pictures of the same period, most but not all of them British, in which photographers represented social distance by the space between the figures in the picture (see Fig. 4.44). It is, however, difficult to know to what use the second American picture could have been put; it may simply have been rejected as a poor photograph.

This was almost certainly the fate of another unconventional picture. In 1904, surgeons who had been trained at the Johns Hopkins Hospital were photographed operating together to celebrate the opening of a new amphitheatre. The surgeons autographed and circulated a souvenir photograph of the occasion which looks much like other pictures of surgery taken at the time (Fig. 3.80). There are, however, other photographs of the same operation which the surgeons did not sign, and which depict surgery in ways that look unusual, notably in the cluttered appearance of the operating theatre (Fig. 1.3). Such unconventional photographs are not necessarily more revealing than the conventional ones. The unconventional image was only an alternative account of surgery which most surgeons did not acknowledge as accurate.

It is very hard, in fact, to know how unconventional photographs were regarded. For example, a house officer in Boston just after the turn of the century took a photograph of a smallpox patient and pasted it in his private casebook (Fig. 3.42). An unconventional image of a nurse was, incidentally we think, framed in this photograph. The image is unconventional because she is not depicted, as nurses usually were at that time, as a neat, tidy presence. Unfortunately, we have no evidence about how contemporaries would have interpreted this image. She might have been seen as tired and dishevelled because of her labors. On the other hand she might have been perceived as slovenly. Context-of-use here is everything.

Similarly, we have a photograph of a man and a nurse in a hospital ward in Boston in the 1890s (Fig. 1.4). We know, from other sources, that the man was a house officer and that the photograph was kept with the private papers of a physician and deposited in an archive by his son.[6] It is tempting to provide an historically unjustified text and to read the photograph as a unique example of sexual interest—to see the house officer staring lasciviously at the nurse. But was he?

It is too easy to give such pictures a modern meaning they were never meant to convey because we do not know enough about a subject. For example, a photograph of black and caucasian patients at a United States Public Health Service clinic in the South in the 1920s was once misinterpreted by the American co-author as a statement about integration in public medical care (Fig. 1.5). Further study suggested, however, that contemporaries may have been expected to see this picture as stigmatizing men of both races who had acquired venereal disease, but perhaps especially the black men who, unlike the whites, stood and faced the camera.

Some unconventional photographs were certainly not the results of accidents. For instance, in 1912 the eminent American surgeon, Harvey Cushing, while on a European study trip, took a photograph of an apparently blood-spattered assistant surgeon which Cushing later placed in his diary (Fig. 3.86). We have seen only a few other photographs from before the 1920s that so vividly represented blood. Before then, surgery was almost always represented as a singularly spotless business. It is probable that there was a private imagery shared by surgeons and another public one.[7] Although it is impossible to know how this picture was read, it is a reminder that surgery, like every aspect of medicine, was almost always photographed with a limited visual language. Similarly, while physiologists were occasionally photographed performing animal experiments, these were usually private records; their public images were almost invariably confined to portraiture.

This book is an account of the photographs of medicine produced in Britain and the United States since the mid-nineteenth century. It is a comparative history for reasons both accidental and historiographic. We studied American and British photographs because we know about the history of medicine in these two countries. However, we are also interested in identifying and explaining similarities and differences in perceptions of medical care. Neither Britain nor the United States was medically homogeneous, however, and an interesting study could be done on differences between states or regions. For instance, we note incidentally to the main theme a number of examples in which medicine in Scotland was represented rather differently from medicine in England.

The next four chapters tell the story of the creation of a distinctive visual imagery for medicine and the meanings of that imagery in America and Britain. Chapter II describes the earliest medical photographs, which are mainly portraits of doctors and clinical pictures. We suggest in this chapter how and why distinctive conventions were eventually made to distinguish clinical pictures from other portraits. We also try to discover how medical portraiture relates to the social position of the profession in the nineteenth century. In Chapter III we look at the dominant medical imagery in the thirty years before World War I. This photography depicted hospitals as caring and custodial institutions. More important, photographs, increasingly, represented surgery and public health medicine as the most progressive medical specialties. Chapter IV deals with the interwar years and suggests that photography was one of the means by which medicine increasingly presented itself as interventive as well as caring. In Chapter V, we examine the relations of medicine and photojournalism, and argue that the most important feature of post-Second World War photography was the centrality of the patient as its subject.

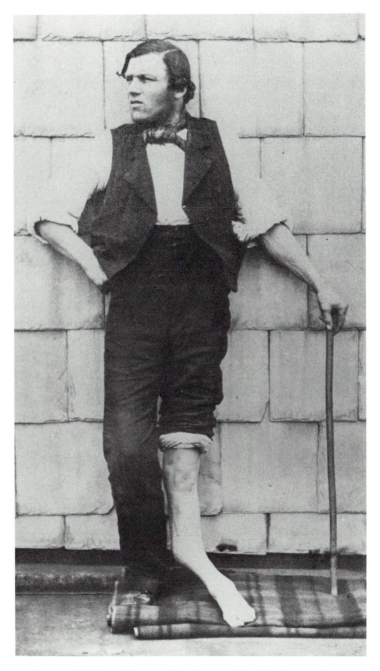

Fig. 1.1 Clinical photograph of an unidentified man, from an album of pathological studies, c. 1865 (The Royal Society of Medicine).

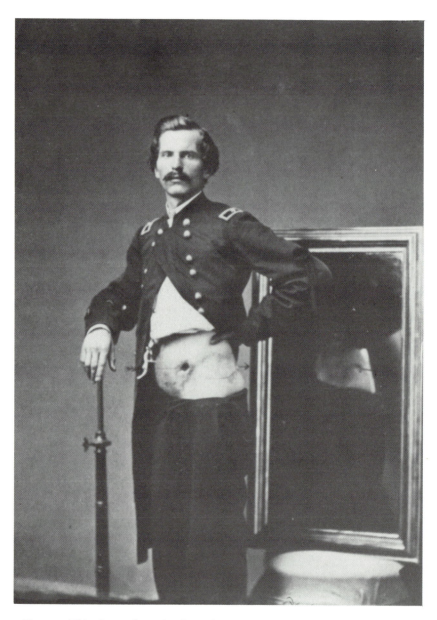

Fig. 1.2 This General received an abdominal wound during the Civil War. The mirror provides a view of the wound. The photograph may have been taken by George A. Otis, Surgeon General of the United States Army, 1875 (National Library of Medicine, from U.S. Army Medical Museum).

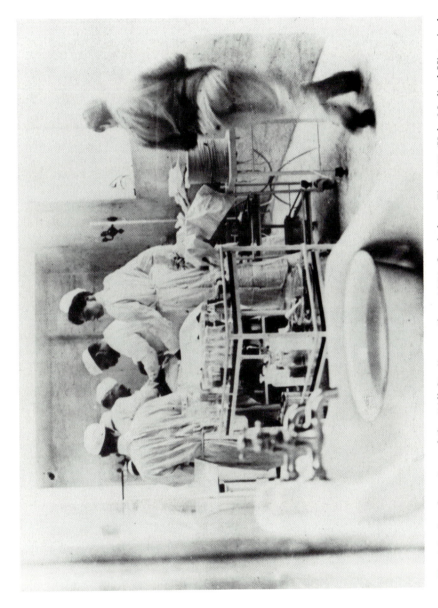

Fig. 1.3 Another view of the "All Star" operation, 1904. See below, Fig. 3.80 (Yale Medical Historical Library).

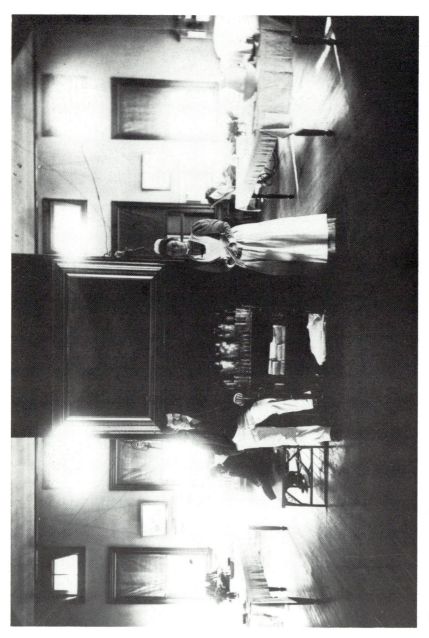

Fig. 1.4 Dr. Arthur Lambert Chute with an unidentified nurse, Boston Lying-In Hospital, c. 1895. The windows in the background were not blacked out, as was customary at the time, which suggests that the photograph was hastily composed (Countway Library, Harvard Medical School—Chute Collection).

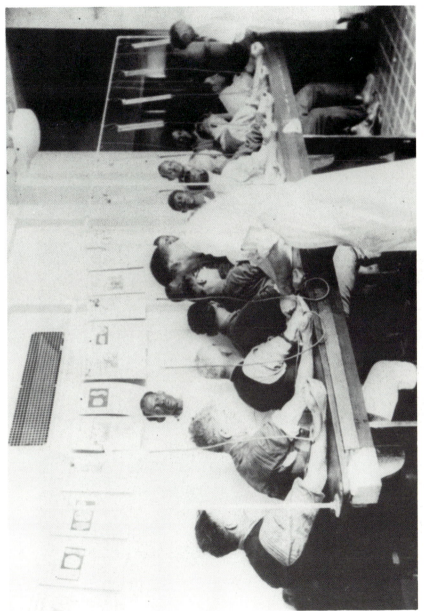

Fig. 1.5 Blacks and whites receiving treatment in the same clinic in the American South, c. 1925 (National Archives of the United States).

CHAPTER II

PORTRAITS OF DOCTORS AND DISEASE, 1840–1890

In the early nineteenth century the collection and recording of facts was generally claimed to be the proper method for acquiring knowledge and thus facilitating progress. Soon after its invention the camera was widely employed in such new disciplines as anthropology and criminology where recording was considered essential.[1] Similarly, within medicine, where claims to scientific expertise and a commitment to measurement and recording became increasingly prominent, the possibilities offered by the camera were quickly exploited. It was only slowly, however, that the medical photograph was transformed into a distinct object. Between the 1840s and the 1890s many of the conventions used in making photographs of medicine were the same as those employed in producing pictures of other activities. Pictures of doctors and of patients looked much like contemporary portraits. Similarly, photographs of anatomical and pathological specimens employed the style of traditional medical engravings. In this chapter, we describe how medical men first used photography. We will analyse some of the earliest photographs of patients and doctors and explore how and why clinical and pathological photography were made distinct from portraiture.

By the mid-nineteenth century, the medical press was an enthusiastic advocate for photography which was, as *The Lancet* put it, "the Art of Truth."[2] From the 1850s onwards British and American medical journals regularly carried general items on photography, reporting for those of their readers who were amateur enthusiasts such technical innovations as the use of magnesium to produce artificial light or the attempt to fix colors.[3] In both countries many hundreds, perhaps thousands, of doctors took photographs either alone or with their companions in amateur photographic societies. They used cameras to represent themselves and their patients and to display pathology.

However, photography did not present medical men with truthful representations the like of which they had never seen before. Quite the reverse: the earliest photographs of doctors, patients or pathological specimens must necessarily have looked to contemporaries very much like accomplished drawings, or like watercolors drained of their tints. Indeed, because the camera incorporated the perspectival rules which had been used in drawings for centuries, photographs could be made into engravings, or conversely, by hand-tinting them, they could be made to resemble traditional colored prints.[4]

Throughout the nineteenth century, doctors in Britain and America were key figures in the history of photography.[5] They participated in the creation of the medium in three ways. As inventors and enthusiasts they helped to improve and popularise the new technology. As members of a rapidly changing profession they used portrait photography to create an image of themselves. As exponents of science, they used the camera to record and define disease.

The standard histories of photography describe the important role of doctors in the creation of the new technology. Among noted photographic inventors were the American physician, Paul Beck Goddard, who, in 1839, described the use of bromine as an "accelerator" and the English physician, Richard Leach Maddox, who, in 1871, announced his discovery of the use of gelatin to bind light-sensitive silver salts to glass and thus create a dry plate. Doctors were also at the forefront of photography as leading photographers of nature and amateur portraitists. The Scottish surgeon, Thomas Keith, for example, produced a now famous series of calotypes of Edinburgh in the 1850s, and the American physiologist, John William Draper, was one of the earliest portraitists.[6]

One of the commonest medical uses of the camera was to produce portraits of doctors. In America and Britain in the early nineteenth century, the middle class appetite for cheap portraiture was an incentive to inventors to try to fix and duplicate the images made by cameras. Middle class demand also provided a ready market for such pictures. Doctors were quick to employ the new technique of self-representation. The majority of medical pictures we have seen from the period 1840-1890 are either individual or group portraits of doctors. In the 1840s medical men appeared in the pictures produced with the relatively laborious and expensive technologies of this era, the daguerreotype and the calotype. In 1854, however, the possibility of public exposure expanded when André Eugene Disdéri patented the photographic *carte-de-visite*, an albumen paper colloid print. These pictures could be produced both cheaply and in great numbers. Many doctors had such cards made (Fig. 2.1). They sent them to their colleagues, exchanged them at meetings and, in England, bought those of famous physicians for a shilling.[7]

By the 1870s, with the appearance of cabinet portraits, pictures of eminent medical men could be purchased serially and also bound in sumptuous biographical works. In Britain the College of Physicians began to keep portraits of its Members and Fellows.[8] With increasing frequency medical men, alone or in groups, appeared in photographs as erudite, dignified pillars of middle class respectability. The profession presented an image of cultured dignity to a public that was still dubious about the claims of medical expertise and progress. In these years medical men often posed with the insignia of academia, a book perhaps, or a gown (Fig. 2.2). The backgrounds which photographers used for making portraits at this time very often represented libraries and never places of medical work. Doctors were rarely photographed with medical instruments although this was not an invariable rule and often in America, sometimes in Scotland, and in one or two instances in England, practitioners posed for portraits with medical or scientific devices (Fig. 2.3).[9]

Nineteenth-century medical men also appeared frequently in group and composite portraits. These were sources of pride and, occasionally, controversy. National and international meetings in particular were occasions for taking such photographs. Photographers, however, sometimes found it difficult to attain the proper representation of medical hierarchy at such events. In 1873, for example, a writer in the *British Medical Journal* criticized a photograph of an annual meeting of the British Medical Association because some doctors "occupy a very prominent place in the foreground while eminent medical men . . . are reduced to physical insignificance in distant corners."[10] Contemporaries, it seems, had observed a rare failure of the "Art of Truth." When doctors considered such pictures satisfactory, for example the massive composite portrait of the 1881 International Congress (Fig. 2.4), they used them to celebrate the uniqueness of medical life.[11] In addition to being photographed as elements of a single profession, doctors who worked in new sciences and specialties, such as experimental physiology, obstetrics or bacteriology, frequently took commemorative photographs of their meetings.

At the same time that doctors and their photographers began to create an imagery of medical men, they also produced new representations of the body and disease. After about 1850, professional journals regularly reported attempts to apply photography to every area of medical interest, including anatomy, physiology, histology, and pathology. Medical societies actively encouraged their members to collect pathological and clinical photographs.[12] The photography of morbid anatomical and microscopical specimens, however, presented problems as well as possibilities, and, at least until the end of the century, doctors often preferred traditional representational techniques, such as engraving.

The visual representation of morbid *organic* specimens rather than of people who suffered afflictions was a relatively new event in the history of medicine. Beginning in the late eighteenth century, notably in France, detecting organic change by physical diagnosis—by looking, listening, touching, and smelling—became increasingly important in medical practice. This creation of a visual concept of pathology occurred at the same time that new technologies—wood engraving, lithography, the steam printing press, and photography itself—made it cheaper and easier than ever before to reproduce drawings of bodily organs in large numbers. By the twentieth century the visual demonstration of disease at post-mortem and in the pathological museum, and its representation in pictures, became central to medical education.

Soon after the invention of the modern camera, doctors attempted to represent morbid anatomical specimens in photographs in the same way in which they were shown in the great pathological atlases illustrated by lithographs or hand-colored engravings.[13] However, the early photographs of diseased organs proved disappointing. Although photography could represent the relative sizes and shapes of pathological specimens, the detail in the pictures was indecipherable. This was because photography did not imitate the conventions which lithographers and engravers employed to distinguish the textures and colors of pathological specimens—cross hatching, for example. Doctors had learned the pathological significance of these conventions from journals and textbooks illustrated by traditional means. In 1886, the author of a paper in the *British Medical Journal*, complaining about photographs of morbid anatomical specimens, revealingly stated that such pictures looked like Ovid's chaos since they "failed to give a good idea of what they are *supposed to represent.*"[14] Photography did not displace drawing to depict morbid anatomy until new conventions were created to represent tissues and tissue change.

Similar difficulties occurred in the interpretation of histological photographs. Around mid-century, pathologists argued over the relative merits of the engraving and the photograph: about their accuracy and their capacity to represent clearly what they wanted each other, and their students, to see through the microscope. An early enthusiast for the use of the camera in microscopy, Lionel S. Beale, wrote, "Very much yet remains to be done in representing microscopic texture faithfully . . . . there must always be many appearances which can only be rendered by accurately copying them by hand."[15]

Gradually, however, histologists and morbid anatomists made photography a useful mode of representation. They devised new ways to prepare specimens and introduced special photographic techniques for producing consistent representations of the features in the specimen the pathologist saw as important. Eventually mass reproduction of such pictures made possible the widespread distribution of statements about the visual characteristics of organic diseases. Such imagery served heuristic purposes in a similar way to that of specialized maps in the new science of geology.[16] They allowed pathologists to see the diseases others had described in the dead, and clinicians to envisage and locate them in the living.

Doctors also attempted to use photography to represent disease in the living. The first photographs of patients were of two sorts: pictures of typical cases of well-known diseases and visual reports of extraordinary abnormalities. Rather later, it was frequently proposed that the clinical photograph should form a routine addition to all hospital patient records. This practice was adopted in some institutions, most often asylums. A parallel usage to this was the regular photographic recording of members of such groups as degenerates, criminals and alcoholics.[17]

Daguerreotypes of patients were taken in the United States in the late 1840s.[18] Shortly after this, many patients were photographed in both countries and hundreds of pictures from the 1850s and 1860s survive. When picturing the sick, the earliest photographers employed the conventions used in making ordinary portraits. In most photographs the patients wore everyday clothes and were surrounded by domestic furniture, both of which gave clues as to their social class and perhaps, therefore, to the diagnosis. This was particularly true of photographs used as typical cases and especially so in the instance of lunatics, whose pictures were frequently taken to demonstrate the general features of different mental diseases. In America in the 1840s, daguerreotypes of convicts were used as the basis for published engravings which were considered to represent the types of moral depravity. In 1852, Hugh Welch Diamond, medical superintendent of the Surrey County Asylum at Twickenham, showed photographs of the inmates in order to illustrate "the *types* of insanity."[19] Many of Diamond's photographs were used as lithographs by John Connolly in 1858 to demonstrate "the physiognomy of insanity." Connolly considered the photographs exact "illustrations of the forms of insanity."[20] Such photographs, because they were portraits, used many of the same clues as hand-made pictures for distinguishing types of madness.[21] Mad men and women, for instance, were depicted with fixed stares, and with their hair and clothes in disarray.

The most frequent subjects of early clinical photographs, however, were people suffering from extraordinary physical illnesses or disabilities. In 1858 *The Lancet*, urging doctors to use the camera more widely, noted "the surgeon employs it but very seldom, and then only to delineate some cases of extraordinary deformity or unusual interest."[22] Many photographs survive of Siamese twins, people with severe deformities, huge tumors, multiple limbs and massive wounds (Fig. 2.5, 2.6, 2.7). Doctors, in other words, had begun to photograph as pathological objects the freaks who fascinated their contemporaries in fairs and circus side-shows.[23] But because such pictures employed the style of ordinary portraiture they created problems, for they did not signal to viewers that these pictures were to be regarded as having medical rather than any other sort of interest. In 1865, for example, the *Lancet* published an engraving, made from a photograph, of a famous contemporary freak, a man with duplication of the genitalia (Fig. 2.8). The picture provoked a response which condemned the use of "physiology . . . as a mere mask for obscenity" and deplored the journal "pandering to the lowest and foulest tastes."[24]

A series of photographs taken by the British physician, Alexander Balmanno Squire, exemplifies many of these points about early clinical and pathological representations. Squire's pictures were produced in book form, between 1864 and 1866, to show characteristic examples of common diseases of the skin. The patients were presented in portraits. The lesions were hand coloured in order to make them look very much like traditional prints (Fig. 2.9). To the viewers, of course, this made them appear more real. Thus the *British Medical Journal* could regard the pictures as "singularly perfect representations of typical cases."[25] Similarly, this American photograph from the 1860s was tinted red to show the blood running from the patient's arm into the bowl (Fig. 2.10).

By the 1890s, because of the establishment of laboratory science and experimental and clinical pathology as the source of medical perceptions, relatively distinctive conventions had been established for producing photographs of the sick. They were made anonymous, often by blacking out the area over and around their eyes. Photographers less frequently recorded clues about social class except when depicting the results of therapy. Subjects were increasingly photographed naked and against plain backgrounds (Fig. 2.11). Often the parts of the body which were not diseased were eliminated from the print (Fig. 2.12).

The capacity to make these representations was partly related to such technical innovations as close-up lenses, the dry plate and improved spectral sensitivity in film. The relationship between technical innovation and changing photographic conventions is complicated, and beyond the scope of this book. Close-up lenses and more sensitive films were available when the distinctive conventions for photographing patients were created; but this is not to say that the new conventions were determined by the technology.[26]

The elaboration of a new visual language for describing the objects proper to medical study also helped to create or to reinforce special areas of expert enquiry. The new conventions defined some subjects which were once matters of everyday public interest as privileged areas of medical knowledge. Freaks, for example, were no longer photographed as curiosities but were depicted as part of the subject matter of a systematic science: teratology.

By 1900, illness in medical pictures had been thoroughly naturalized as pathology. The conventions used in portraiture no longer had a place in pictures taken to record and display disease and its results. The conventions of clinical photography were further changed during the twentieth century, corresponding to changing medical perceptions. These changes probably did not involve the same sort of major reorientation in disease representation as occurred in the nineteenth century. The history of these changing conventions of clinical photography and their relationship to technical innovation in both photography and medicine deserves careful study. For the purpose of this book, however, we ignore the history of clinical photography after it became a specialized practice rarely visible to the public. During the twentieth century, the imagery of medicine visible in the public sphere ceased to be combined with the specialized imagery of disease.

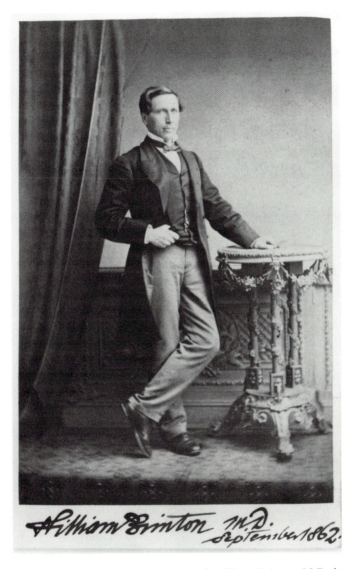

Fig. 2.1 Carte-de-visite portrait of William Brinton M.D. by
C. T. Newcombe, London, dated by hand September 1862. 9 × 6
cm. Brinton was a Fellow of the Royal College of Physicians,
England, and a physician at St. Thomas's Hospital, London
(Wellcome Institute Library, London).

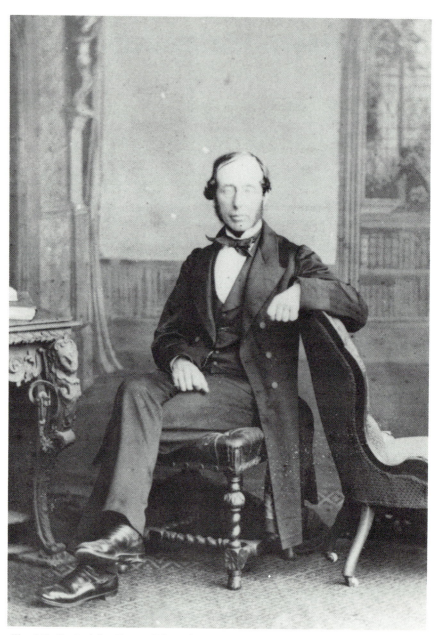

Fig. 2.2 Portrait by Ernest Edwards, London, of the Dublin physician William Daniel Moore in W. T. Robertson (ed.), *Photographs of Eminent Medical Men* (London: John Churchill, 1868, Vol. 2, facing p. 115) (Wellcome Institute Library, London).

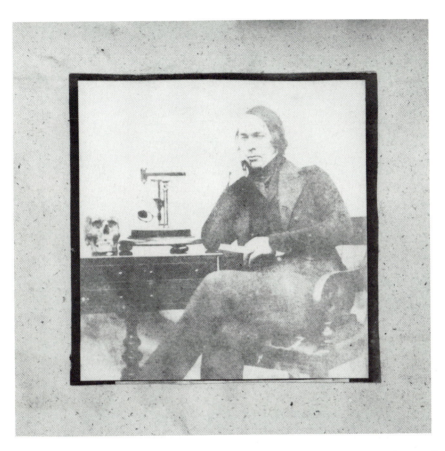

Fig. 2.3 Calotype of John Reid, 1842. Reid was a physician and a professor of anatomy, which explains the presence of a skull. His interest in the basic sciences probably accounts for this picture of him with a microscope (National Museums of Scotland, 1942—5576).

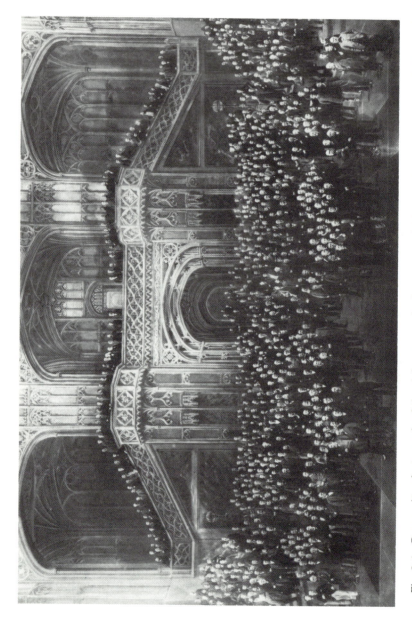

Fig. 2.4 Composite photograph of the delegates at the International Medical Congress 1881 by G. Barraud, n.d. (Wellcome Institute Library, London).

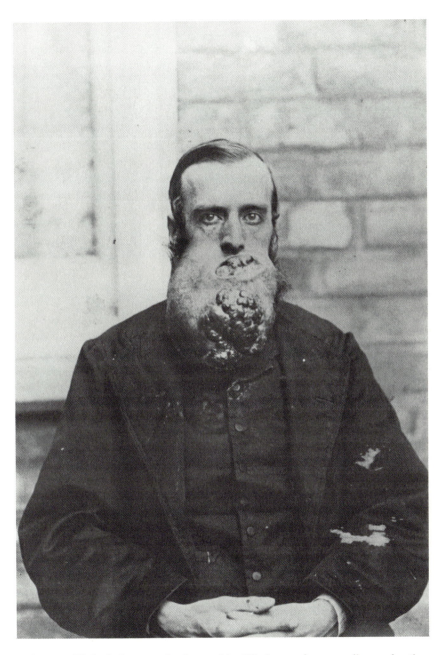

Fig. 2.5 Clinical photograph of an unidentified man, from an album of pathological studies, c. 1865 (The Royal Society of Medicine).

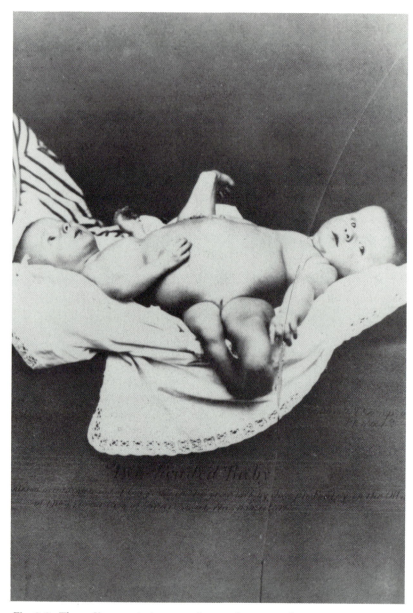

Fig. 2.6 These Siamese twins, age six months, were photographed, c. 1870, by the firm of Gihan and Thompson for one of the early books of photographs of medicine and surgery, Louis A. Duhring and Francis Fontaine Maury, eds., *Photographic Review of Medicine and Surgery* (Philadelphia: J. B. Lippincott and Co., 1871-1872).

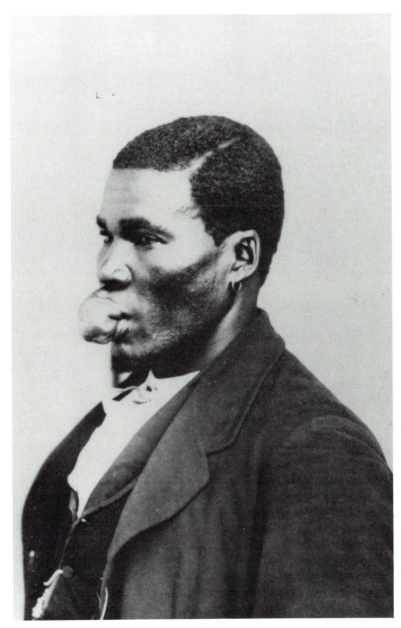

Fig. 2.7 A man with a venous facial tumor, c. 1870. The patient wore street clothes and the side of the face with the tumor was turned away from the camera, perhaps in order to contrast it with the patient's normal aspect. Louis A. Duhring and Francis Fontaine Maury, eds., *Photographic Review of Medicine and Surgery* (Philadelphia: J. B. Lippincott and Co., 1871–1872).

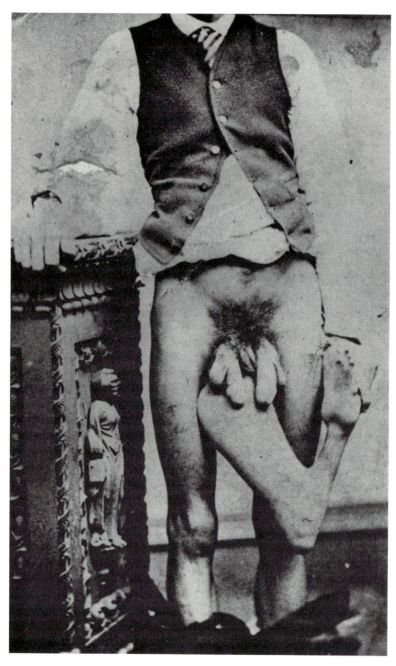

Fig. 2.8 The famous "freak" Juan Dos Santos, from an album of pathological studies in the Royal Society of Medicine, c. 1865 (The Royal Society of Medicine).

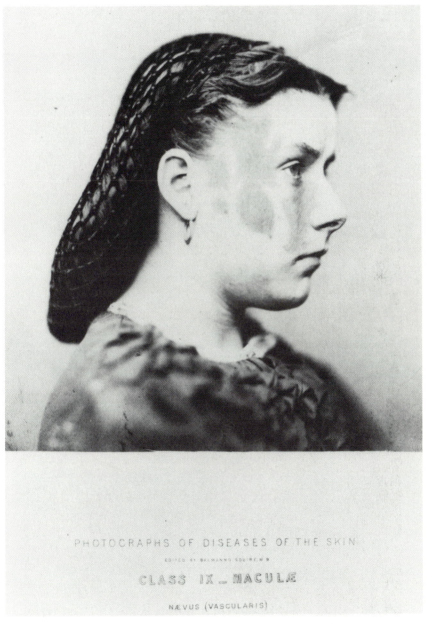

PHOTOGRAPHS OF DISEASES OF THE SKIN

EDITED BY BALMANNO SQUIRE M.B

CLASS IX — MACULÆ

NÆVUS (VASCULARIS)

Fig. 2.9 From A. J. Balmanno Squire, *Photographs (Coloured from Life) of the Diseases of the Skin* (London: J. Churchill, 1865) (Wellcome Institute Library, London).

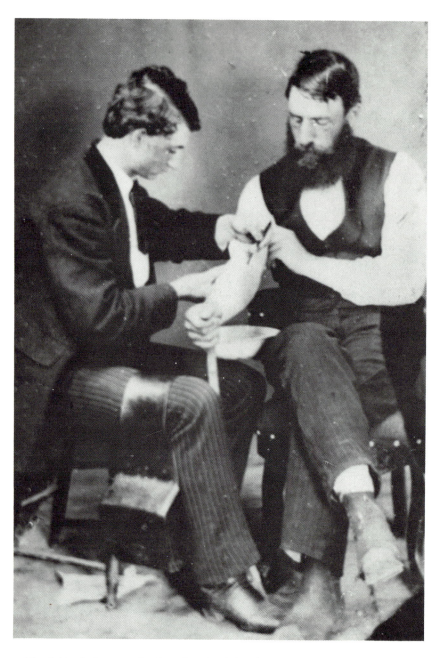

Fig. 2.10 A tintype of a frontier physician letting blood, c. 1860 (Stanley B. Burns and the Burns Archive).

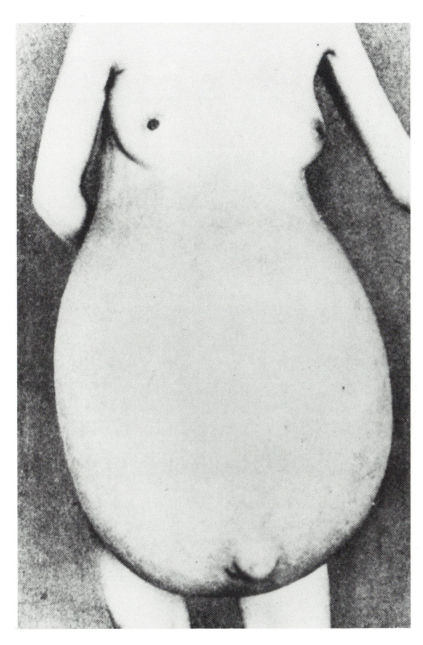

Fig. 2.11 A uterine tumor, c. 1900. Contrast this photograph with Figs. 2.6, 2.8 and 2.9. Harold Speert, *Iconographia Gyniatricia: A Pictorial History of Gynecology and Obstetrics* (Philadelphia: Davis, 1973).

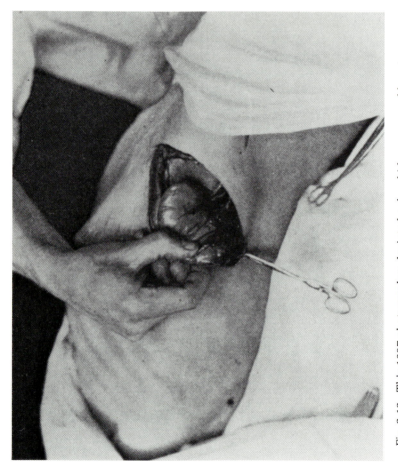

Fig. 2.12 This 1897 photographer depicted only a kidney, exposed by a transverse incision on an abdomen, a surgeon's hand and forearm and two instruments. N. Senn, *Tuberculosis of the Genito-urinary Organs, Male and Female* (Philadelphia: W. B. Saunders, 1897).

CHAPTER III

DEFINING AN IMAGE, 1880-1918

In the four decades before the First World War, more photographs were taken in hospitals than in any other medical arena. Doctors and governors (called trustees in America) commissioned photographs of most aspects of hospital life for reports, postcards and commemorative albums. Wards were the most frequent photographic subject. We chose two pictures to describe the conventions of ward photography in America and Britain in these years. Figure 3.1 is representative of many British voluntary hospital images of the period. It is a postcard, made from a photograph taken in 1899 of a ward in St. Bartholomew's (Bart's), a London teaching hospital. Figure 3.2 was taken in the 1890s at Bellevue Hospital in New York City, a municipal institution which received charitable contributions and also had teaching responsibilities.[1]

Consider the postcard from Barts. At a quick glance, it resembles a picture of a Victorian home. The room contains such common domestic objects as plants, a mirror, a rug and an easy chair. In other ward photographs from these years there are paintings, pianos and, on rare occasions, a parrot (See Fig. 3.29). But the postcard also shows that the room was not in a private home and that its purpose was not merely domestic. The photographer chose an angle of vision that emphasized the high ceiling and the light entering from the tall windows. The electric lights, which must have been a recent installation, were also included. Perhaps to attract the viewer's gaze to the long sink at the end of the room, the photographer let his own image be reflected in the mirror beneath the window. At the left and right of the picture, patients, hospital staff, and plain metal beds are in an orderly arrangement.

Furthermore, even though there are reminders of domesticity in this picture, the people do not behave as they would in family photographs of the time. They are distant from each other. The patients lie or sit staring straight ahead. The nurses stand, not engaged in any obvious work. In this ward a clergyman is prominent. Pictures of hospital chapels were very common at this time.

Although differing in detail, many British ward pictures from the decade before the turn of the century have an overall appearance similar to this one. Pictures of Poor Law hospital wards are rarer, but not so very different.[2] In some photographs domestic furnishings are more, in others less, abundant. At times doctors pose in the spaces between beds and furnishings. The nurses are sometimes seated and often they hold a child. Almost all these photographs suggest—as do contemporary written sources—that the people responsible for British hospital pictures attempted to create an image of the hospital centered on the ward, which was the focus of a clean, well-ordered, benevolent, pious and caring institution. In such places, medical intervention was subordinate to domestic order.[3]

Figure 3.2 differs from the photograph of Barts, in part because Bellevue was a municipal institution rather than a voluntary hospital, but also because medicine was often visualized differently in the two countries. Like the ward at Bart's, it is neat and brightly lit. Although the ward was most likely about the same size as the one at Barts, it seems to be more spacious. Moreover, there are no domestic objects in the room: everything has an obvious medical use. The focal point of the picture is a simple clock at the center of the rear wall of the ward. In contrast to the British photograph, two doctors are present. Moreover, both of them, together with nurses, are occupied with patients. In this, as in many other American photographs of the time, wards were places in which medical work was done. Even twenty years earlier, American wards do not seem to have been represented in quite the same way as wards in Britain. In the 1870s, for example (Fig. 3.3), a ward at Bellevue was photographed as a specialized work setting. This difference between the photographs taken at Bart's and at Bellevue makes plain that the conventions of hospital pictures were not determined entirely by what the camera could do. People in British hospitals were not photographed standing and looking at the camera merely because of the limitations of photographic technology. It was perfectly possible to produce pictures of people at work.

Private rooms in American hospitals in the 1890s, in contrast to their spartan wards, were depicted as more luxuriously domestic than any general hospital interior in Britain (cf. Figs. 3.4 and 3.5).[4] By the early twentieth century, however, private rooms in most American hospitals seem to have been photographed to resemble miniature wards—unique settings for medical care that also assured privacy to those who could afford to pay (Fig. 3.6).

Not all photographs of British wards taken in the 1890s had a domestic appearance, and increasingly after this time, photographs from the two countries looked very similar. By 1910 domesticity had all but disappeared from photographs of general hospitals. The origins of this change in British ward photographs were complex, but they included the supplanting of the lay control of hospitals by medical men, especially surgeons. The result was an imagery that represented British general hospitals as places of medical work. The children's ward in the newly opened Birmingham General Hospital in 1897 (Fig. 3.7), appeared to be far more spacious and empty than the ward at Bart's, although the rocking horse, the plants and the furniture would still have reminded the Victorian viewer of domestic life. In contrast, a photograph of a children's ward at the Massachusetts General Hospital taken at about the same time (Fig. 3.8) would have looked to contemporaries very much like one of an adult ward. Not surprisingly, given the demands for recognition made by fringe medical groups, this picture of the interior of the Homeopathic Hospital in London used the imagery of orthodox medicine (Fig. 3.9).

In chapter I we noted that doctors and nurses in large hospitals in the United States frequently appeared in photographs which resembled middle class family portraits (Fig. 3.10). The middle class home may also have been the model for describing at least some types of work done in American hospitals. For instance, nurses were frequently depicted working alone, much as housewives actually did. Other aspects of American hospital work were photographed in much the same way as they were in contemporary industrial establishments.[5]

In Britain, by contrast, representations of upper class homes seem to have supplied the conventions for photographing large hospitals well into the twentieth century. The hospital was often depicted as a great country house, complete with its gatekeeper (Fig. 3.11). Hospital staff usually sat for group portraits in the grounds of the institution rather than within it (Fig. 3.12). On the wards they maintained a distance from each other appropriate to their stations (Fig. 3.13). The staff were divided into a downstairs class, in the kitchens and the laundry (Fig. 3.14), and an upstairs elite, the doctors, (Fig. 3.15) with porters (Fig. 3.16) as go-betweens. Even the pharmacy (Fig. 3.17) seems to have been photographed to look like the brew-house of a manor, not, as in America, like a shop for making and dispensing drugs (Fig. 3.18). Moreover, in Britain, women were rarely photographed working, and hardly ever working alone.[6] Photographs taken in small British hospitals, on the other hand, often depicted the staff as close families.

In both countries, although patients frequently were represented in photographs, they were usually incidental elements in pictures about other matters. With the exception of children they were rarely given prominence as individuals or depicted in a relationship with other people. British patients were often represented waiting in grand institutions (Fig. 3.19), almost always in the presence of figures of authority. American photographs of waiting patients were composed in the same way (Fig. 3.20). The existence of a large number of photographs showing poor people waiting for medical attention suggests that such pictures had important meanings for contemporaries. They may have been read as evidence of the efficiency of medical philanthropy, or of its heavy workload. Such pictures, when used to advertise the hospital, undoubtedly signalled that it was proper for the poor, in both countries, to be patient and obedient when visiting the hospital. Much less frequently, photographs represented charity care as compassion for the helpless. These objects of charity were often children, as can be seen in this unusual Scottish picture from 1910 (Fig. 3.21).

Photographs taken in small or specialized hospitals frequently incorporated different images from those we have described. A picture of a battlefield hospital in the American Civil War can be contrasted with the many photographs of long, neat wards in military hospitals behind the lines. It may have been taken to portray the difficulties of providing medical services at the front (Fig. 3.22). That it was carefully constructed for a purpose is suggested by the lack of blurring in an era when exposure time required patience on the part of the subjects. Photographs of improvised hospitals might also have been used to represent order or containment as in this example from a set of pictures taken in the 1890s of a Gloucestershire hospital for victims of smallpox (Fig. 3.23). Many small, special, and local British hospitals advertised their "cottage" image rather than the domesticity of a great house. In both Britain and America, photographs of hospitals for people suffering from chronic or incurable diseases usually showed a home-like environment (Fig. 3.24).

Pictures of sanatoria for the tuberculous only occasionally contained people who appeared sick. The most frequent photographic subjects were the restorative benefits of open air and the companionship of fellow sufferers (Fig. 3.25).[7] Photographs of interiors were rare, except when they suggested access to the out-of-doors. A British photograph, for instance, showed how a Mediterranean climate had been institutionalized for the benefit of consumptives in Greater Manchester (Fig. 3.26). A composite photograph of an American patient before and after a stay in a sanatorium (Fig. 3.27) advertised that the treatment had improved his tailoring and his social life. Occasionally sanatorium photographs did not conform to this pattern. Some people, perhaps patients themselves, seem to have taken pictures to show that life in these institutions was tedious and lonely (Fig. 3.28). Sanatoria patients were almost the only hospital inmates before World War I to be photographed in a style resembling that used for portraits. Patients with tuberculosis were accorded special status in photographs, just as they were in fiction, poetry and painting.

British asylums, both public and private, were usually depicted as domestic—sometimes luxuriously so (Fig. 3.29). Nearly all the British photographs of such institutions taken before World War I portrayed large, self-sufficient country households. Colney Hatch Asylum produced a portrait of its attendants dressed in smart uniforms (Fig. 3.30). In contrast, the custodial activities of British asylums were not represented. Instead, mental hospitals were shown as places in which staff cared for the helpless patients while the other patients looked after themselves and the asylum (Fig. 3.31). Group portraits of patients, at rest, work, or recreation, were common and were presumably taken to show that asylums were places where people were happy to live. An unusual set of photographs were taken of the Scottish asylum, Sunnyside, at Montrose, by an employee, W. C. Orkney, who was also an amateur photographer. In addition to producing conventional pictures of communal labor for the benefit of the institution (Fig. 3.32), Orkney made arresting studies of patients which show them as individuals. Presumably the mad, like patients with chronic tuberculosis, had a different photographic status from the acutely ill poor (Fig. 3.33).[8]

American asylum photography was very different from British. Although Americans occasionally photographed mental hospitals as great country estates and depicted patients doing menial work, they frequently depicted asylums as medical institutions where doctors and nurses used technology to diagnose and manage patients (Fig. 3.34). Moreover, unlike the British, Americans occasionally represented the custodial role of the asylum, for instance the use of restraint (Fig. 3.35). We do not know, however, the context in which this photograph was used.

There were differences in the photography of hospitals in the two countries, but in both nurses were essential to the images. Like patients, nurses were usually shown on the wards as anonymous figures (Fig. 3.36). As we have seen, nurses in British hospitals were hardly ever photographed at work, even of the most polite sort. Unconventional photographs were presumably taken for private use (Fig. 3.37). In neither country do representations of nurses include blood, sweat, and tears, let alone pus, urine or faeces, which we know from other sources were a constant presence on hospital wards. The representation of spilled body fluids and excretions was not permissible in the late nineteenth century, except in a limited number of contexts, such as heroic painting. It was certainly not conventional in hospital pictures. These photographs signalled moral and material order rather than the presence or threat of disorder.

American hospital nurses, unlike those in Britain, were often depicted in multiple roles. They were shown at work, consistent with the common representation of the hospitals as sites of medical activity. Many photographs showed nurses caring for small children in images that combined the familiar features of order and work (Fig. 3.38). They were photographed receiving classroom education (Fig. 3.39).[9] They were also, but only occasionally, shown as privately employed in homes (Figs. 3.40, 3.41), which was, in fact, where most trained nurses in America worked in this period. There were also unusual representations of nurses. One example, which we noted in Chapter I, was taken by a house officer in Boston just after the turn of the century. He photographed a nurse with a drawn face and disordered hair (Fig. 3.42). At Montrose, W. C. Orkney produced a portrait of a nurse in an uncommon pose in which he drew attention to her expression. This was, we know, a private picture (Fig. 3.43).

In both countries, a uniform was the defining convention that made a woman a nurse, whether in portraits, off duty, on the wards, in the classroom or in the home (Figs. 3.44, 3.45, 3.46, 3.47). Doctors, on the other hand, were identified by the whole range of conventions employed to photograph men and women of the educated classes (Fig. 3.48).

Probably only a few photographs of British senior medical men on the wards or in outpatient clinics were taken before the First World War (Figs. 3.49, 3.50). Most British physicians and surgeons were photographed outside hospitals, usually in portraits. This doctor's private consulting room was represented as a genteel study (Fig. 3.51).[10] Britain's most illustrious hospital physicians and surgeons chose to be photographed holding their canes (Fig. 3.52). In contrast, many American academic doctors had themselves photographed using the stethoscope (Fig. 3.53), or instructing students beside a patient's bed. However, photographs of British hospital practitioners who graduated around the turn of the century began to include diagnostic and other technology. One such physician (Fig. 3.54) drew attention to his stethoscope. A thermometer and temperature charts were also prominent in the composition.

The education of new practitioners was not photographed in the same way in the two countries. Gross anatomical dissection, although regarded on both sides of the Atlantic as the foundation of medical education, was depicted rather differently. Official American pictures of gross anatomy laboratories are common and similar to some contemporary images of factories (Fig. 3.55). This stark image of efficiency was, however, often subverted by American students, who routinely took commemorative photographs of themselves posing with cadavers (Fig. 3.56). In Britain on the other hand there are only a few private photographs of dissecting rooms and published images are very rare (Fig. 3.57). This published photograph of a dissecting room with cadavers was used to convey a complex message about the conflicting demands of military recruitment and medical education (Fig. 3.58).[11]

Photographs of medical students being taught in laboratories were taken in both countries, although much less often in Britain. American medical schools often used pictures of their laboratories to advertise their modernity. British photographs seem to have been taken for individual use, for example, this picture, which is unusual because it is an early representation of women medical students (Fig. 3.59).

Americans regarded clinical education as a significant photographic subject and represented it frequently. Many photographs survive of groups of students surrounding a teacher and a patient in hospital wards, clinics, and lecture rooms (Figs. 3.60, 3.61). In contrast, when British students appeared in photographs, they were usually incidental to the main subject of the picture (see above Fig. 3.49). Unlike most American students, moreover, they were often photographed in casual poses in clinical settings. Photographs, then, were another one of the ways in which medicine was defined as a technical occupation by Americans and as a genteel vocation by the British.

Most doctors, of course, did not see patients in teaching hospitals. After qualifying, the majority of doctors had little further contact with elite hospital medicine and usually practiced from rooms (called surgeries in Britain) in their own homes. Although there are numerous literary idealizations of British general practitioners and a number of dramatic representations of them in paintings and engravings, as far as we can ascertain there are no photographs of them at work in their surgeries.[12] They were, of course, photographed in family portraits, as fathers and husbands. There are at least two possible reasons, not mutually exclusive, why there was no imagery of the British general practitioner. First, the control of medical imagery lay elsewhere, in the hands of consultants and in the hospitals rather than among isolated general practitioners. Second, these practitioners were advertising that their relations with their patients were sacrosanct. This seems likely in view of the importance they attached to being photographed *outside* their surgeries. For example, they often had pictures taken while they went on their rounds in their carriages (Fig. 3.62), and some years later, very many more were photographed in their cars, often with a chauffeur (Fig. 3.63).[13] In this unique and undecipherable pair of photographs, a rural general practitioner is shown as a landed sporting gent in the humble task of tooth-pulling (Figs. 3.64, 3.65).

By contrast, for reasons that are not clear, many pictures survive of American doctors in their offices. The only ones which include patients seem to have been taken in small towns, perhaps because the doctor and patients were also being depicted as friends and neighbors. In the mid-1890s, for example, a doctor in Wichita, Kansas, was represented treating a patient while other people sat in the same room. The office was shown as a parlor, with domestic wallpaper, wall hangings and lighting (Fig. 3.66).

Patients, however, were usually not included in photographs of doctor's offices. A doctor in Minneapolis, Minnesota, in the late 1890s was photographed reading in his office (Fig. 3.67), which was quite unlike a parlor. The photographer chose an angle of vision which emphasized the objects in the center and at the right of the room. A glass case of medical tools, a functional metal lamp and an examining table dominate the picture. The photograph incorporated an uncarpeted floor and light-colored walls, on which hung what the contemporary viewer would probably have assumed were the doctor's credentials and a medical group portrait.

It seems that American doctors who treated the urban elite only rarely permitted their offices to be photographed (Fig. 3.68). This picture, taken of a Boston physician's office in 1914, has more in common with the British photograph of a consulting room (Fig. 3.51) than with other American portraits of doctors' offices. The doctor was depicted as both a gentleman and a man of science, working in a room that looked like one in a well-furnished home. The photograph included medical instruments, a uniformed nurse and the doctor wearing an examining mirror. To the right, an examination couch was depicted; it resembles domestic furniture, rather than the functional, purpose-built, examining table in Fig. 3.67. The doctor displayed not only domestic and scientific objects but also his works of art: a winged statue, two pictures of what appear to be classical scenes, and a drawing or a photograph of the Rialto.

The juxtaposition of science and domesticity may have been appropriate for an elite Boston practitioner, but, by this time, American hospitals were increasingly representing themselves as centers of applied science. This transformation occurred in Britain but more slowly and unevenly. In both countries, however, by 1910 photographs began to show clinical pathological laboratories (Fig. 3.69), radiology rooms, and pharmacies rather than kitchens and laundries. In particular, pictures of technology and, increasingly, of surgery seem to have been offered as examples of the importance of science in medicine.

Until the 1920s the new medical technology that was appearing in both British and American hospital photographs was not represented in any consistent fashion. Machines were sometimes photographed among familiar domestic objects. Here, for example, a Roentgen Ray apparatus sat among potted plants (Fig. 3.70). In an unusual British picture, an early electrocardiograph was shown with a white coated technician (Fig. 3.71). It is unusual because such ancillary staff were rarely photographed and white coats were only occasionally sported as hospital uniforms. Nurses were often photographed simply sitting alongside machinery, perhaps in the same way that earlier pictures had depicted them holding or watching children (Fig. 3.72). It was the technology itself, not the space in which it was being used, that was important in all these early British pictures. Later, the site where the technology was used—X-ray rooms, for example—became the photographic subject. In

America, similarly, conventions for photographing technology were only gradually established. This early photograph that seems today to depict a randomly cluttered room, may have been used to display the complexity of new equipment (Fig. 3.73). The people using the new technologies were, at first, displayed in various ways; sometimes watching, but occasionally working. In some American pre-war photographs, medical staff were no longer represented in pictures of therapy based on elaborate technology (Fig. 3.74).

More important, however, beginning in the late nineteenth century the number of photographs of surgery greatly increased. By 1914 surgery was represented by a totally new set of conventions. In the earliest photographs of surgery (Figs. 3.75, 3.76), practitioners, patients and observers wore street clothes and performed operations in wards or in plain rooms or, during wars, in ordinary tents (Fig. 3.77). Familiar domestic objects, such as jugs, basins, and buckets often appeared in pictures of surgical procedures. Separate operating rooms existed at this time, but they were rarely photographed.

During the 1880s in America, surgery in the photograph changed. The group around the patient became smaller than in the past, people began to dress distinctively and each had a visible role. This is evident in a picture of surgery on a ward at Bellevue in the late 1880s (Fig. 3.78). Each of the four surgeons and three nurses performed a task. The vessels on the floor were grouped in an orderly relation to the operating table and the nurses. Yet there were also older elements in this photograph: for instance the patterned window curtain, another patient in a bed, and the plant at the lower right. Surgery was still represented as an activity in a public place.

By the 1890s, the way in which surgery was usually photographed, especially in America, had been more precisely defined. Written sources attest that surgeons began to perceive operations as rituals. The British surgeon, Berkeley Moynihan, was said to have approached every operation as a "religious rite or sacrament."[14] The representation of such a ritual can be seen in a photograph taken in 1888 in the recently opened amphitheater for the abdominal ward of the Massachusetts General Hospital (Fig. 3.79). Nursing students observed from above; and two other observers, a physician and a nurse, stood to the right. A third observer, the only one in street clothes, stands behind the principal surgeon, who seems to handle a tumor removed from the patient. Each of the other surgeons performed a task. Again, older elements persisted: ordinary buckets were in the left foreground and the patient's foot protruded from the sheet.

Surgeons increasingly regarded operating as a performance. One particularly splendid enactment was the reunion of eminent surgeons to perform what they called the "All Star" operation, which we described in Chapter I (Fig. 3.80). The conventions that were used to depict such performances were also employed in photographs of less august surgical occasions. Charles H. Mayo, for example, was photographed in 1911 operating at St. Mary's Hospital in Rochester, Minnesota (Fig. 3.81). The photographer stood to the right and at a higher level than the operating table. Mayo was in the left foreground and the surgeons watching were reflected in the mirror above him. No part of the patient was visible.

The changing photography of surgery was integral to the revolution during which surgeons made themselves the most vigorous of the medical specialists. Surgeons increasingly regarded and represented themselves as distinctive, because of recent advances in science and surgical technique.[15] They were, one of them boasted in 1905, "apart from and above" their colleagues; creators of "miraculous" and "increasingly marvelous" works.[16] Surgeons presented this new self-image in the photographs they displayed to themselves, to other doctors and to the general public. Thousands of photographs represent surgeons *apart from* other doctors and other areas of the hospital. Many photographs presented them as *above* other doctors or as the focus of their attention; these images were often described by contemporaries as heroic.

Most historians have used these photographs only as a record of surgical change. This approach to these sources separates photographs from the social process by which they were made. Photographs were part of the transformation of surgery. They can be used to establish detail about past surgical practices; but to use them exclusively for such a purpose is to ignore their historical context.

By the beginning of this century British surgery, like surgery in America, was often photographed as a special performance with a central figure (Fig. 3.82). British surgeons, however, never created so vivid a verbal or visual language of heroism as their American colleagues. In contrast to America, for example, photographs did not show large audiences arranged in tiers in amphitheaters. From the end of the 1890s, however, surgical theaters, often empty, were regularly photographed in Britain (Fig. 3.83). By the time of the First World War hospitals were producing postcards of surgical operations. Indicative of the prestige of surgery, the techniques which made it distinctive—sterilization for example—were depicted prominently in other hospital photographs (Figs. 3.84, 3.85).

The new imagery of surgery, it should be noted, was defined as much by what was ignored as by what was included. In the first chapter, we described a photograph, taken by Harvey Cushing in 1912, which depicted blood (Fig. 3.86). Blood must have been part of the visual experience of all surgeons, and yet it rarely appeared in photographs. Somewhat earlier, in 1875, Thomas Eakins *painted* a picture of heroic surgery, *The Gross Clinic*. Unlike contemporary photography, Eakins' painting vividly depicted blood, in red, of course (Fig. 3.87). This painting was hung in the Centennial Exposition in Philadelphia in 1876 where it could be seen by a medical audience.[17] It was not exhibited in the public gallery.

Eakins' picture, we suspect, was used as the model for an unusual photograph of surgery taken in Philadelphia. In 1899, a prominent Philadelphia surgeon was photographed during a surgical demonstration at Hahnemann Hospital (Fig. 3.88). Like Gross in the painting, he dominated a picture in which the figures were arrayed in a pyramid. Like Gross, moreover, he turned toward the spectators who sit on ascending benches which entirely fill the background. The assistants in the right foreground also were arrayed in a way that resembled those helping Gross. Most important, his hands and the surgical sheet seem to be covered with blood.

With limited exceptions the representation of blood does not seem to have been acceptable in photographs of hospital medicine. We have already suggested that representing it would have contradicted the image of cleanliness and order which characterized photographs of hospitals. After all, in a black and white picture, blood is indistinguishable from dirt.

If the representation of dirt was interdicted in portrayals of the hospital, it was, by contrast, essential to many public health pictures. In the 1890s many photographs linked insanitary streets, inadequate sewerage and slum housing with poverty and disease. Alongside this imagery, which was produced mainly by journalists, philanthropists and social reformers, was another which represented a medical remedy for disorder. This was an imagery of active intervention.

This imagery, which appeared in the first decade of this century, supplanted an older public health imagery of regulation and environmental control. Photographs in this latter style had depicted the containment of disease by quarantine (Figs. 3.89, 3.90). Many more advertised the protection of the people's health by the inspection of food and housing, the collection of refuse, and the preservation of public order (Figs. 3.91, 3.92).[18] Others were used to criticize inadequate sanitary facilities (Fig. 3.93). The provision of fresh water, the elimination of sewage and the laying out of parks and gardens were shown as laudable civic ends (Fig. 3.94), as was the establishment of public bathhouses and urinals, photographs of which are common in the archives of British local authorities and the records of American governmental and philanthropic organizations (Fig. 3.95).

Around 1900, however, a new imagery relating to the protection of the public's health was produced. It is clear from other sources that this imagery was, in part, associated with national concern about the physical fitness of the population, especially children. Some groups concerned about degeneration used portrait photography for eugenic purposes.[19] Photographers also recorded the disciplined exercise which was often advocated as the cure for national enfeeblement. During and after the Boer War, for instance, when the British were intensely anxious about the physical condition of the country's youth, photographs frequently represented children exercising at school in military fashion (Fig. 3.96). Group exercise was also photographed in America (Fig. 3.97), but more often to promote self-help programs or to celebrate immigrant traditions. Also, in both countries, group exercise was also shown as an integral part of medical care, especially for chest diseases (Figs. 3.98, 3.99).

This new imagery, however, was also part of a new definition of medicine's role and responsibility in public health. Just as photography was integral to the surgeons' new construction of their place in medicine, so, in public health, it was used by both doctors and nurses to redefine their work as active intervention, using scientific methods to protect individuals. These doctors and nurses, unlike their hospital counterparts, were identifiable by what they did rather than by where and how they stood or sat or by their dress. In the new public health pictures, doctors touched patients or listened to their chests through stethoscopes, and nurses talked, touched, weighed and recorded. In the United States, doctors were photographed examining immigrants as they arrived (Fig. 3.100). In both countries, in the same years, numerous photographs showed members of the poorest classes, especially children, awaiting or undergoing medical inspection (Figs. 3.101, 3.102).

These public health pictures are quite striking for several reasons. Doctor-patient encounters were represented far more often than they were in hospital medical practice. These encounters were depicted as occurring in large public spaces which often included many onlookers. The people in the encounters, moreover, were usually children and immigrants. Their lower socioeconomic and, therefore, photographic, status made it possible to represent their examination as consistent with the *public* good.

Women wearing uniforms were frequently depicted as the providers of education and therapy for injuries and ailments in public health clinics (Fig. 3.103). In the United States, such women also appeared in photographs instructing patients in homes and places of work (Fig. 3.104). Rearing children had become an important subject in both American and British medical photographs. Numerous photographs represented efforts to improve the health of mothers and babies. The pictures of the people who taught British and American mothers how to look after their children showed them dressed in uniforms resembling those worn in hospitals (Figs. 3.105, 3.106). About this time weighing scales began to appear with regularity in pictures showing mothers and babies (Fig. 3.107).

There is a strong contrast between these public health photographs and those taken in hospitals in the same years. Although many of British nurses' activities in contemporary hospital life were never pictured, their colleagues in schools and public clinics were depicted as working women. In the United States, and occasionally in Britain after the turn of the century, numerous photographs were taken of nurses providing care in settings other than clinics (Figs. 3.108, 3.109). The doctors who were photographed in the British local authority clinics were general practitioners who were never photographed in their own surgeries. General practitioners in these clinics were shown at work using instruments and often wearing white coats (Fig. 3.110).

In both countries, but particularly in Britain, the poor were represented as deferential when they received public attention. In Fig. 3.111 authority was ranged on one side of a table, and the respectful poor, at a distance, on the other. The American counterparts of these photographs were pictures of physicians practicing among the urban poor. By the early twentieth century, however, some of the photographs of physicians treating patients in public clinics were composed and captioned in order to dramatize personal stories about the participants. For example, in a photograph from New York City in 1910 captioned, "Tongue Out," a physician examined a child while two women looked on, one a nurse, and the other presumably the child's mother (Fig. 3.112).

In the years before the First World War, then, changes were occurring in the photography of hospitals and public health activities. Those who produced these photographs were creating a visual language which increasingly represented medicine as the effective application of science. By World War I, moreover, patients were beginning to be represented as participants in medical encounters. During the war many photographs were composed in this way.[20]

Many wartime photographs represented the levels of what contemporaries conceived of as hierarchies of science-based military medical care: emergency treatment in the trenches (Fig. 3.113); transportation to casualty clearing stations behind the lines (Fig. 3.114) where surgical skill was mobilized (Fig. 3.115); moving patients to hospitals for specialized surgery and other procedures (Figs. 3.116, 3.117, 3.118); and eventually rehabilitation in military hospitals at home. These photographs represented the hospital as the appropriate site of most medical treatment, and reinforced the pre-eminence of surgery in the visual imagery of medical effectiveness.

The domesticity of early British hospital photographs is strikingly absent in pictures of wartime medicine. The wards in military hospitals were depicted as entirely functional (Fig. 3.119). Functionalism was not, however, a necessary consequence of military life. Rather, it was a result of the dominance of surgeons, and thus of their self-image, in the organization of medical services for the wounded. It would be wrong to assume, however, that the exclusion of domesticity from military photographs was meant to signal impersonal relationships between patients and staff. At the turn of the century, domestic imagery was associated with entirely formal representations of patients and hospital staff. In the new imagery of the war, however, the subject of the picture was often a particular wounded soldier, even when the medical activity was sophisticated surgical intervention for a specific lesion. Patients' faces, for instance, were included in numerous pictures in which they were incidental to the medical theme. Moreover, photographs frequently showed informal contact between hospital staff and the wounded. In this picture, a nurse lit a patient's cigarette (Fig. 3.120).

These soldiers were among the first patients in medical photographs to be accorded personality. They were presented neither as examples of a curious disease, as in early clinical photographs, or as mute recipients of charity. The conventions for representing patients in public health clinics and hospitals were quite inappropriate for depicting men who had new status as heroes (Fig. 3.121). Changing concepts of disease may also have played a part in the formation of this new imagery. In some branches of medicine, for example cardiology and psychiatry, there was a movement away from regarding specific lesions as a sufficient definition of disease and toward a concern with the relationship between particular pathology and an individual's capacity to lead a normal life.[21]

This new interest in people was accompanied by an expanding definition of the subjects that were regarded as legitimate for medical photographs. During the war, American and British hospital nurses were almost always pictured in the midst of some activity and involved with their patients (Fig. 3.122). They were women at work and at war. Many photographs of surgery at the front depicted human beings under stress rather than impersonal ritual. For example, Hugh Cabot, a noted American urologist, was photographed close to a patient after a gas attack (Fig. 3.123). The meanings of such pictures could, however, be thoroughly modified by the context in which they were used. An orderly, for example, interviewed a wounded soldier (Fig. 3.124). The caption under the photograph in an anti-war book a decade later suggested a meaning which was almost certainly different from what originally would have been read in the photograph. A close-up photograph of an amputee lying in bed, surrounded by medical equipment, makes the same point in another way (Fig. 3.125). Was the soldier grimacing in agony or trying to laugh or was he asleep? Such questions only serve to emphasize the ambiguities of a particular photograph. This does not mean, however, that it is impossible to generalize about the meaning to contemporaries of the thousands of photographs which exist of medicine in war. Most of these pictures would have been read as messages about the effectiveness and compassion of medicine.

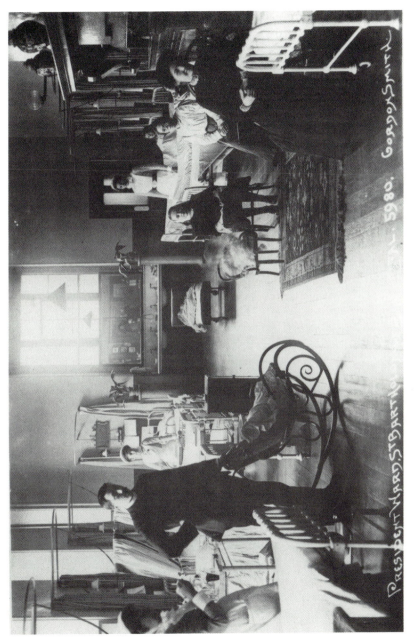

Fig. 3.1 Postcard of President Ward, St. Bartholomew's Hospital, n.d., c. 1899. The photograph makes the ward appear small, yet it contained 24 beds (Wellcome Institute Library, London).

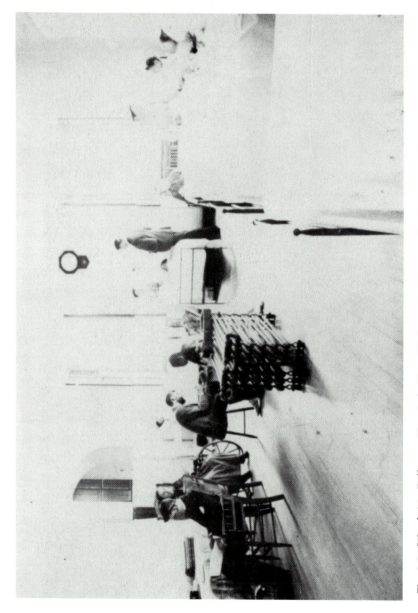

Fig. 3.2 Ward 20, Bellevue Hospital, New York, 1890 (New York University Medical Center Library—012C.c9; also Lady Board of Managers' Collection, Bellevue Hospital Center Archives).

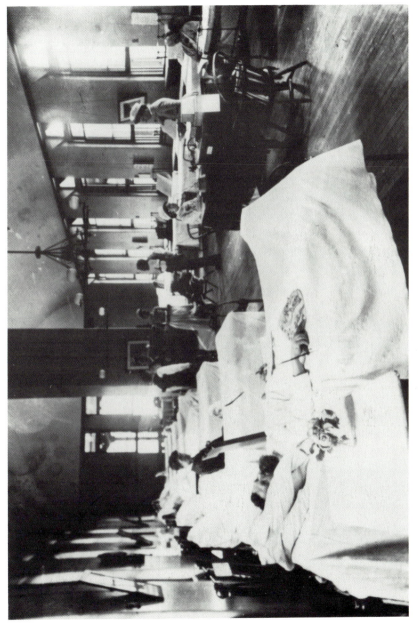

Fig. 3.3 Patients and staff in a ward at Bellevue, c. 1875 (New York University Medical Center Library—012.C.c5).

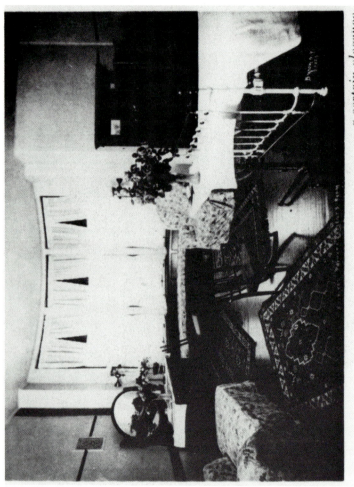

ROOM IN PRIVATE PAVILION—1896

—a certain elegance.

Fig. 3.4 The original caption makes plain the interest of Roosevelt Hospital in New York in recruiting paying patients (United Hospital Fund of New York).

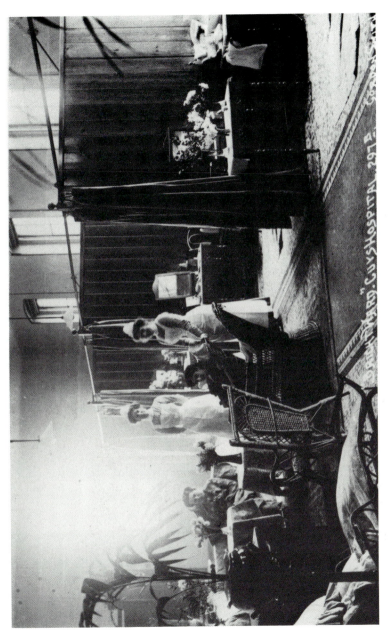

Fig. 3.5 Postcard of Bright Ward, Guy's Hospital, post-marked 1902. The cubicled ward for paying patients was represented in much the same way as the ward at St. Bartholomew's (Wellcome Institute Library, London).

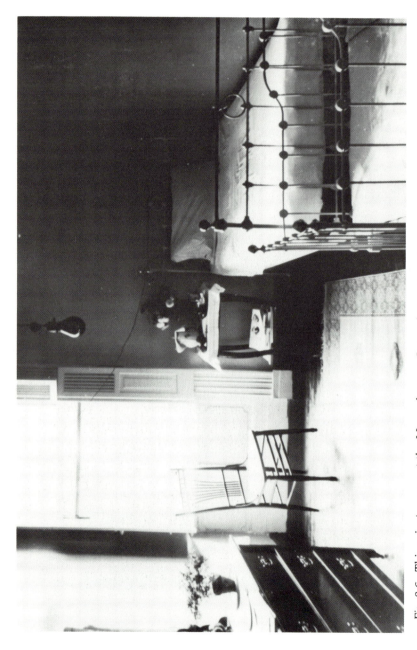

Fig. 3.6 This private room at the Massachusetts General Hospital, photographed c. 1910, was more austere than the one in Fig. 3.4 (Smithsonian Institution, National Museum of American History, Medical Sciences Division—77-5515).

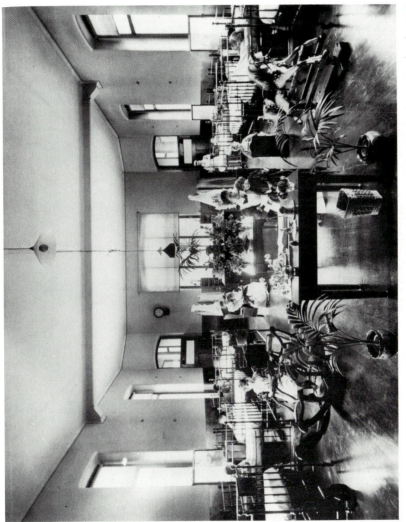

Fig. 3.7 A children's ward in the newly opened General Hospital, Birmingham, England, 1897. The effect of spaciousness has partly been produced by including the ceiling in the picture. It is absent from Figs. 3.1 and 3.5. Note that a clock, as in the functional American ward (Fig. 3.2), has also been included. From a commemorative album (Birmingham General Hospital).

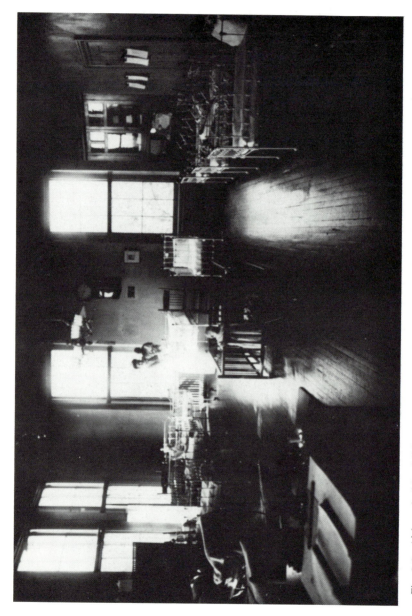

Fig. 3.8 Although this children's ward at the Massachusetts General Hospital resembled an adult ward, the nurse in the middle-ground held a child in the pose conventional for representing pediatric care, c. 1910 (Medical Sciences Division, National Museum of American History, Smithsonian Institution—77-55).

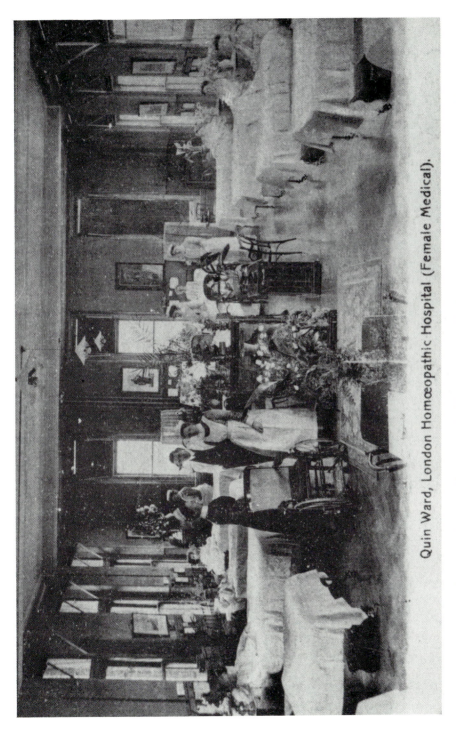

Quin Ward, London Homœopathic Hospital (Female Medical).

Fig. 3.9 A postcard from the London Homeopathic Hospital, c. 1905. It is a typical image of the period. The ward is a comfortable and semi-domestic place, but it is primarily a *medical* institution (Wellcome Institute Library, London).

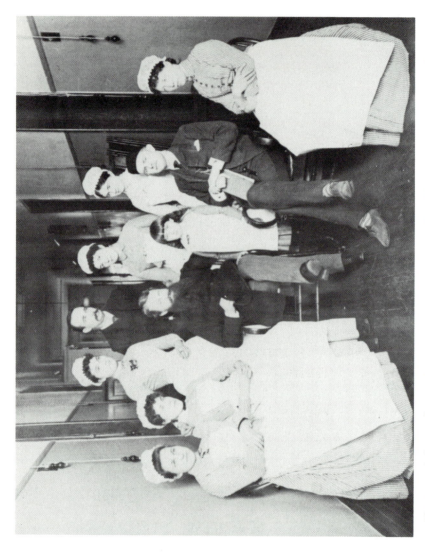

Fig. 3.10 A hospital "family" in a corridor at Boston City Hospital, c. 1880-1890. Compare with Fig. 3.21 (United Hospital Fund of New York).

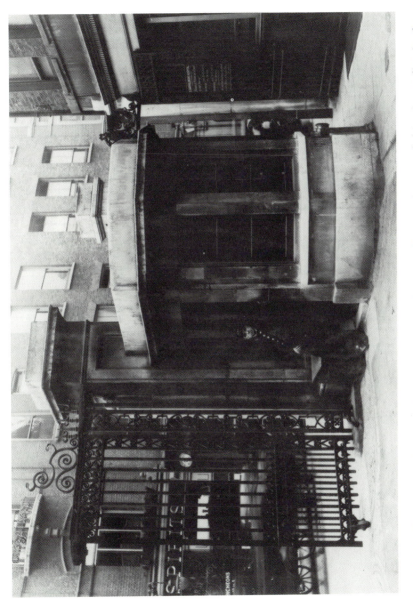

Fig. 3.11 The gates of St. Bartholomew's Hospital, London. The significance of this picture lies in the choice of the gatekeeper as a subject. It has been composed such that the hospital gate is closed against a shop sign advertising spirits (Wellcome Institute Library, London).

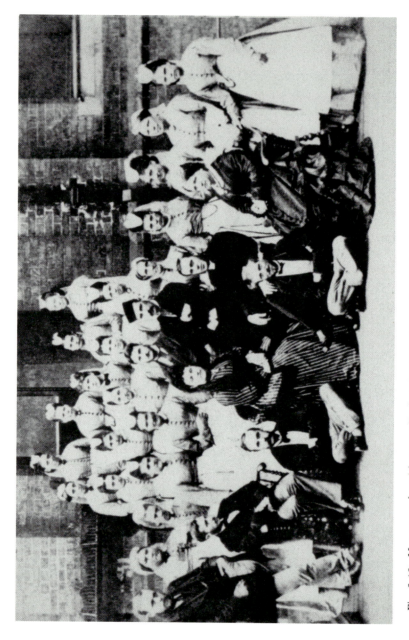

Fig. 3.12 Nurses and resident medical staff of the Leeds General Infirmary, 1874. Group photographs of the staff of country houses, posed in the grounds, were quite common at this time. Note the clergyman is prominent in the composition (Leeds General Infirmary).

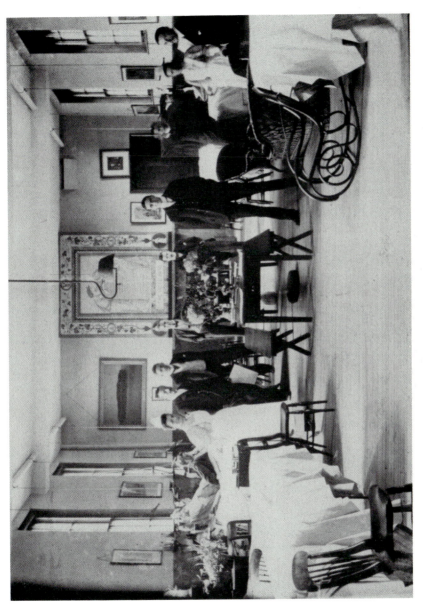

Fig. 3.13 Doctors and nurses in a ward in University College Hospital, London, 1897. From an album in the hospital. Unlike Fig. 3.1, this picture may have circulated only in private (The Library, University College Hospital, London).

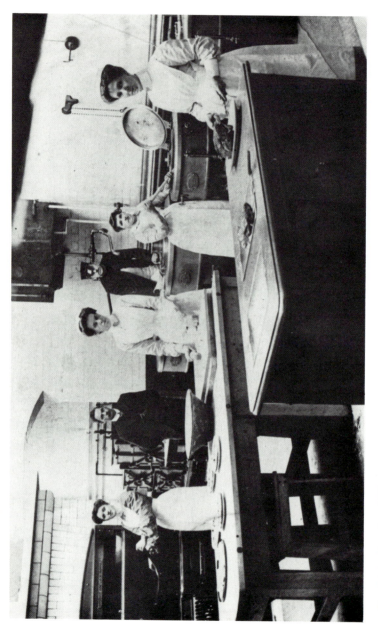

Fig. 3.14 Stepping Hill Hospital, Stockport, England, 1901—the kitchen. Note once again the appropriate distance. The uniformed women and man all handle domestic articles. This, among many other clues, would have shown the contemporary reader that the suited man was the supervisor. Photographs of the kitchens of country houses are very similar in composition (The Documentary Photograph Archive, courtesy of Mr. Hooley).

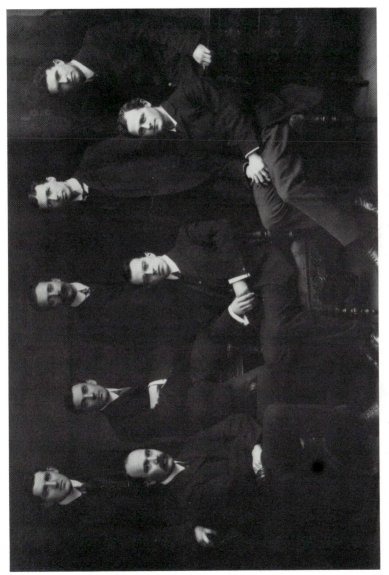

Fig. 3.15 House-surgeons at Charing Cross Hospital, London, 1906. From the album of Dr. Basil Hood, physician at the hospital. Compare this rather ordinary group portrait of young men with the next picture and with Fig. 3.30. All three are typical of the many photographs that depicted hospital staff as loyal and proud members of great institutions (Wellcome Institute Library, London).

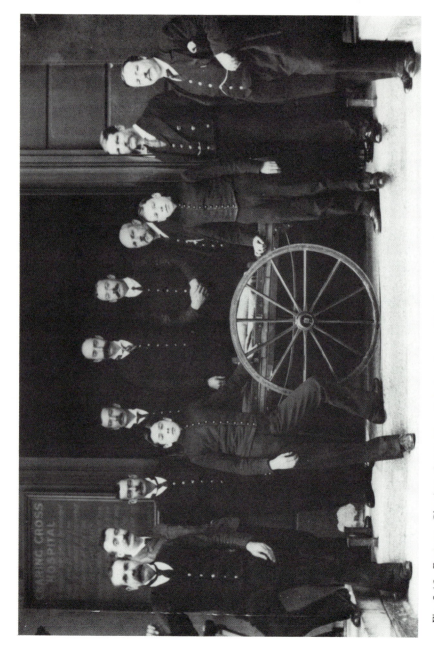

Fig. 3.16 Porters, Charing Cross Hospital, London, 1906, from the album of Basil Hood (Wellcome Institute Library, London).

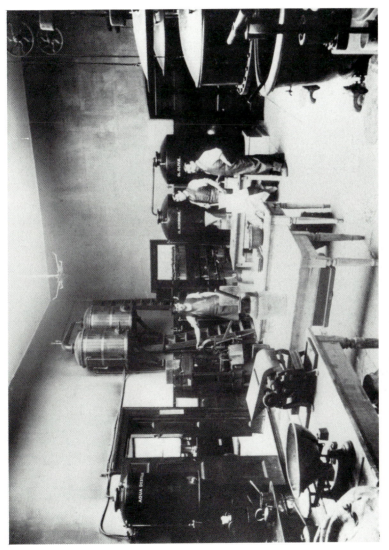

Fig. 3.17 Pharmacy, St. Bartholomew's Hospital, c. 1900. From the hospital archives. This picture is not unlike other British photographs of small workplaces of the time, which contrive to suggest informality and industry. The regimentation found quite early in factory photographs is missing (Department of Medical Illustration, St. Bartholomew's Hospital).

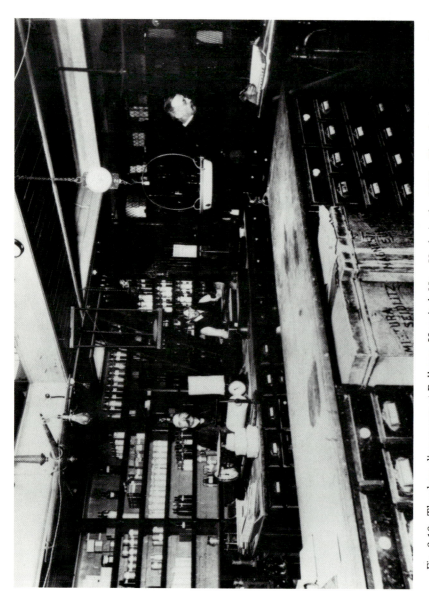

Fig. 3.18 The drug dispensary at Bellevue Hospital, New York, in the 1890s. The photograph resembles those taken of commercial pharmacies in these years (University of Wisconsin-Madison, F. B. Power Pharmaceutical Library—neg. 97734-C-2).

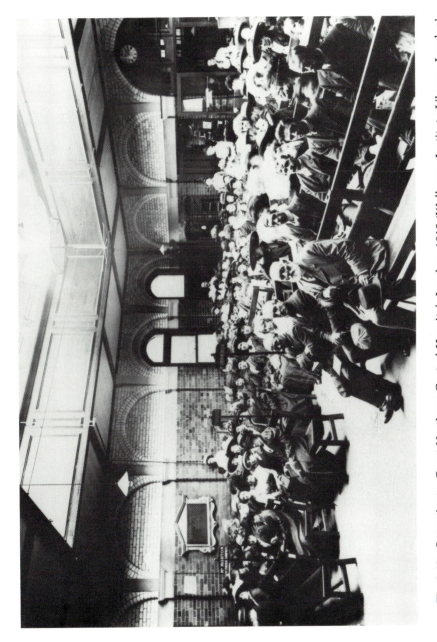

Fig. 3.19 Outpatients, Great Northern Central Hospital, London, 1912 (Wellcome Institute Library, London).

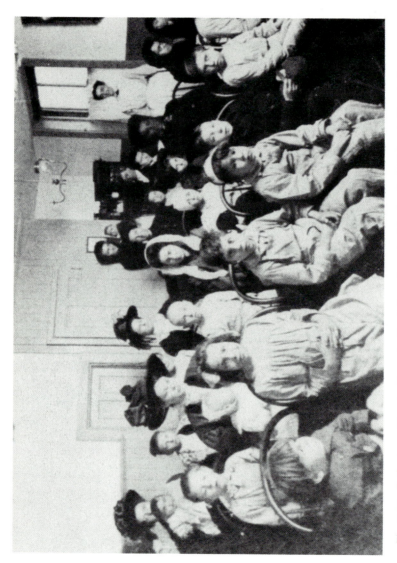

Fig. 3.20 Patients waiting in the outpatient department of St. Louis Children's Hospital, c. 1890. The nurse at the upper right was the American counterpart to the British figures in Fig. 3.19. Although the girl in the front row is large in relation to the other figures in the picture, the composition is not a portrait (Washington University, School of Medicine Library, St. Louis, Missouri—80-9868).

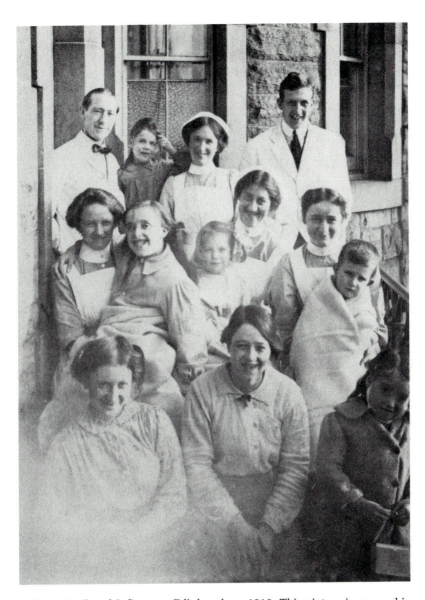

Fig. 3.21 Royal Infirmary, Edinburgh, c. 1910. This picture is unusual in several respects. It is more like a picture of an intimate family than is usually found in photographs from large hospitals. It contains both patients and staff, closely grouped. The impression of familiarity is enhanced by their being photographed smiling. Moreover, it is surprising to find doctors in such an intimate photograph, even if at the rear and above the other figures. Their familiarity is offset by their white coats, also an unusual feature in photographs of the time, although probably less so in Scotland than in England. That the patients are children, and possibly subnormal, may have endowed them with a different photographic status (Royal Infirmary of Edinburgh— R10730/23).

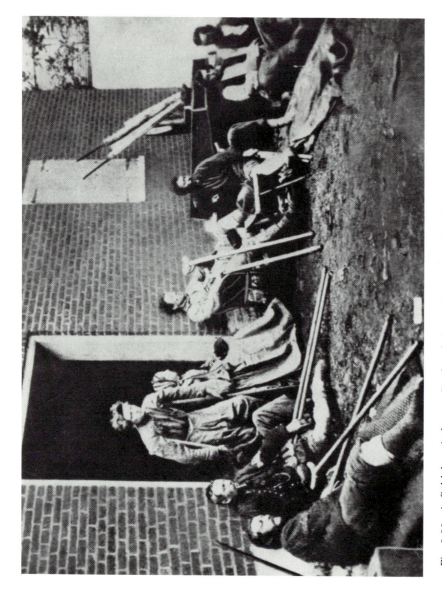

Fig. 3.22 A field hospital near Fredericksburg, Virginia, 1864 (National Library of Medicine—neg. 67-617).

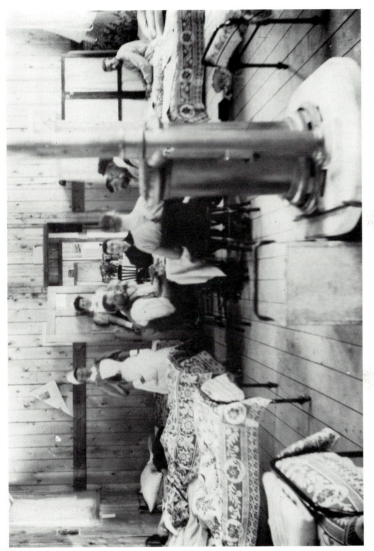

Fig. 3.23 Photograph of a small-pox ward taken in Gloucestershire during a small-pox outbreak in 1886. This picture is contained in an album comprising close-ups of the victims depicting the various stages of their illness. There is circumstantial evidence that it was taken to demonstrate the adequacy of the isolation hospital. Antivaccinationists had accused the authorities of running dirty, over-crowded hospitals (Wellcome Institute Library, London).

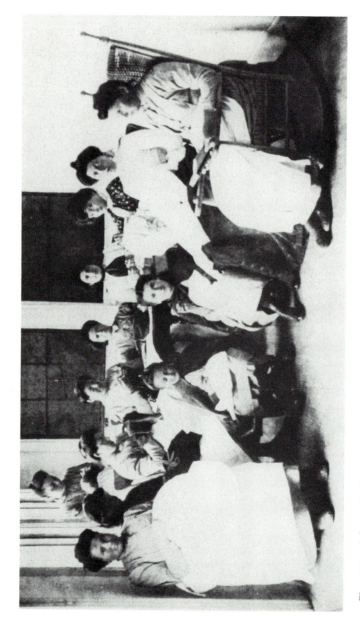

Fig. 3.24 A branch of the Montefiore Home for Chronic Invalids in New York in the 1920s (Montefiore Medical Center).

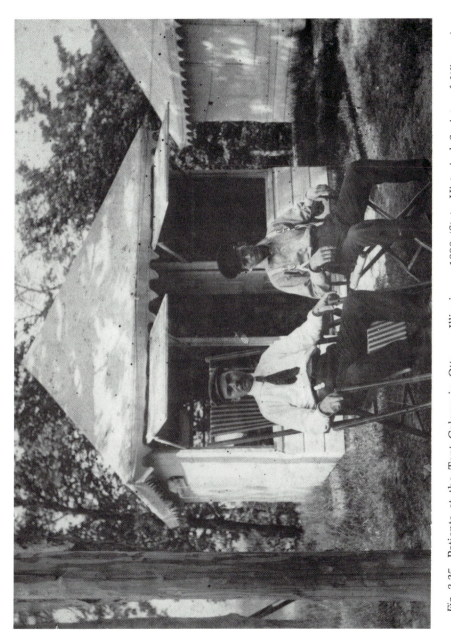

Fig. 3.25 Patients at the Tent Colony in Ottawa, Illinois, c. 1890 (State Historical Society of Wisconsin. American Lung Association—Wisconsin Collection).

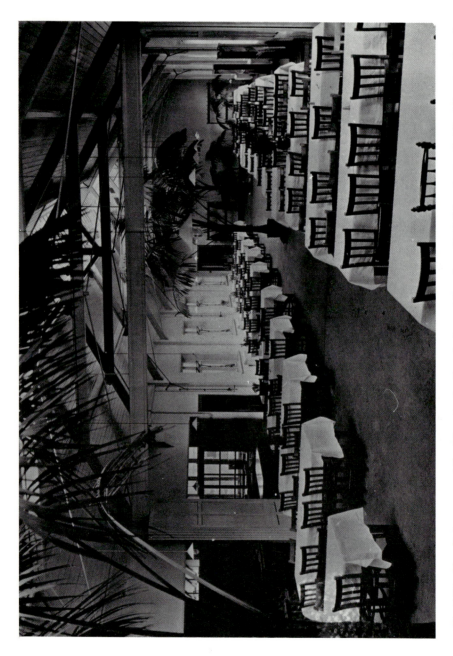

Fig. 3.26 The dining room of the Manchester Sanatorium at Baguley, 1916 (Manchester Public Libraries: Local History Library).

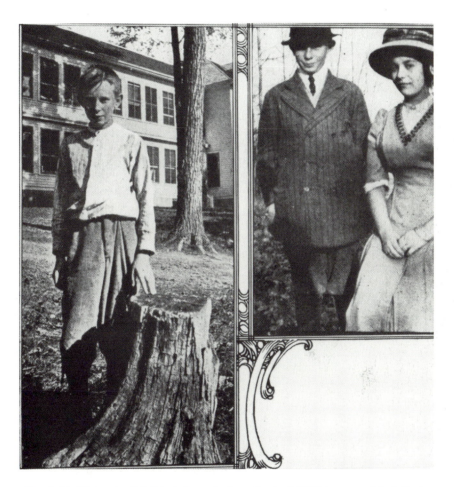

Fig. 3.27 Not only did this tuberculosis patient of 1912 improve his tailoring and get the girl, he was also photographed without the county tuberculosis hospital in the background (*The Journal of Outdoor Life*, 1912).

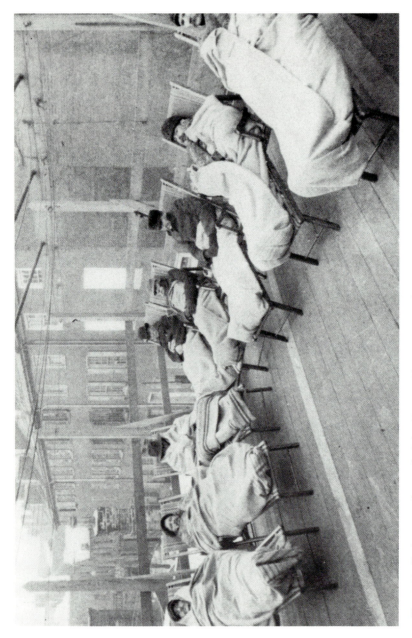

Fig. 3.28 Patients on the roof of the House of Mercy Home for Consumptives, Philadelphia, Pennsylvania, c. 1905 (F. P. Henry, ed., *Founder's Week Memorial Volume.* Philadelphia: F. A. Davis Co., 1909).

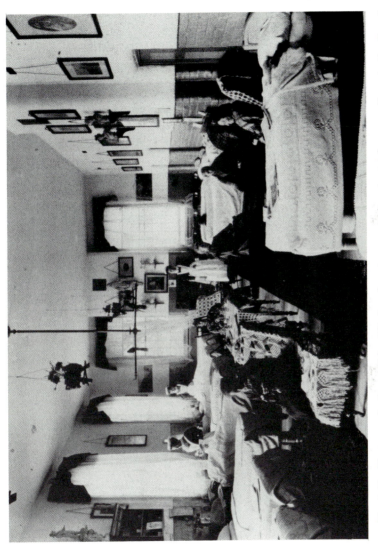

Fig. 3.29 Photograph of an unidentified asylum (presumably private) from an album in the Royal College of Psychiatrists, London, c. 1895. We reproduce this picture as a representation of luxurious domesticity, but photographs from public asylums are compositionally quite similar. For a rare exception, see Richard Hunter and Ida Macalpine, *Psychiatry for the Poor* (London: Dawsons, 1974), p. 157, but we doubt the dating of this photograph as 1900 (Royal College of Psychiatrists).

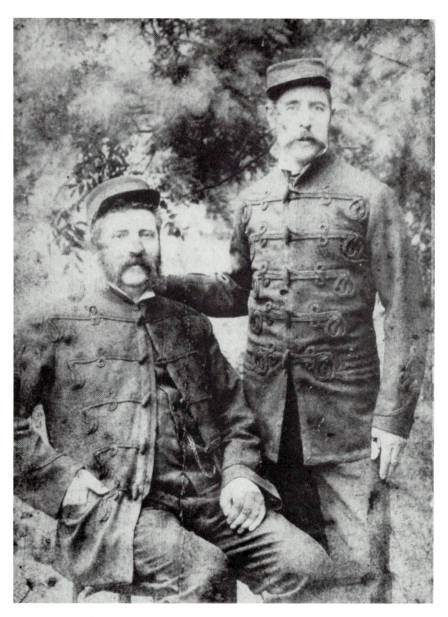

Fig. 3.30 Male attendants, Colney Hatch Asylum, England, c. 1865? (Friern Hospital).

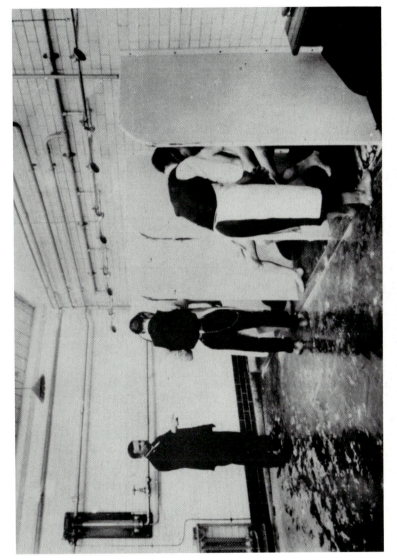

Fig. 3.31 Long Grove Asylum, Epsom, England, c. 1910. From a photograph album in the Royal College of Psychiatrists. On the back of the original is written "The was regarded as an improvement on the old slipper baths." A contemporary reading of this picture, we suggest, would be of institutional care and concern *not* of spartanness and lack of privacy (Royal College of Psychiatrists, original untraceable).

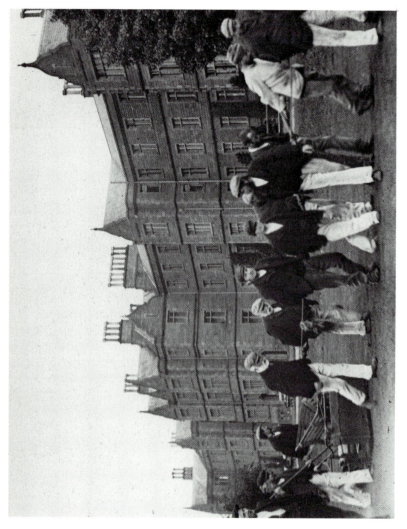

Fig. 3.32 The "mower gang," Montrose Asylum, n.d., by W. C. Orkney. Many similar pictures exist of patients in asylums, working in laundries, leatherwork shops, etc. (Courtesy of the Angus Unit of the Tayside Health Board and Mr. Tom King, Medical Illustration Department of Dundee University).

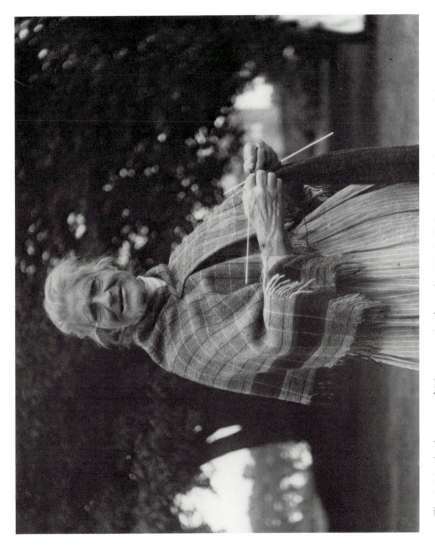

Fig. 3.33 An inmate of Montrose Asylum, by W. C. Orkney, n.d. (Courtesy of the Angus Unit of the Tayside Health Board and Mr. Tom King, Medical Illustration Department of Dundee University).

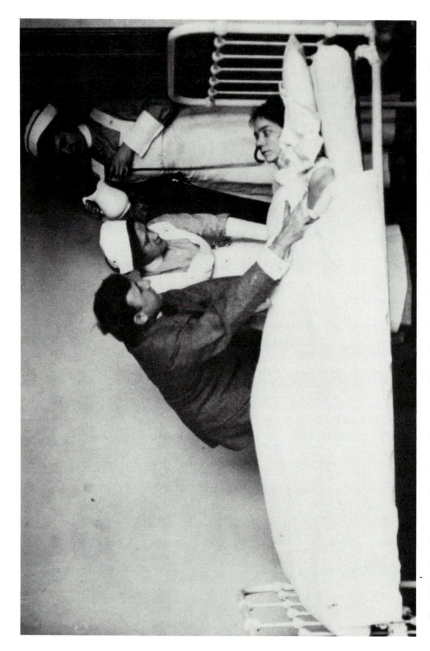

Fig. 3.34 Feeding a patient through a tube, Columbus State Hospital, Columbus, Ohio, c. 1912 (Ohio Historical Society).

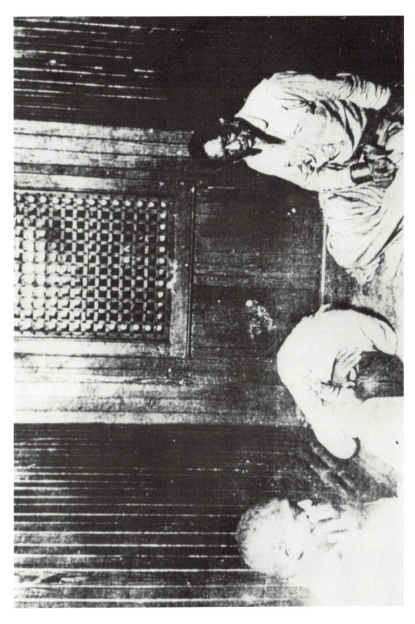

Fig. 3.35 Patients at Dayton State Hospital, Dayton, Ohio, c. 1915 (Ohio Historical Society).

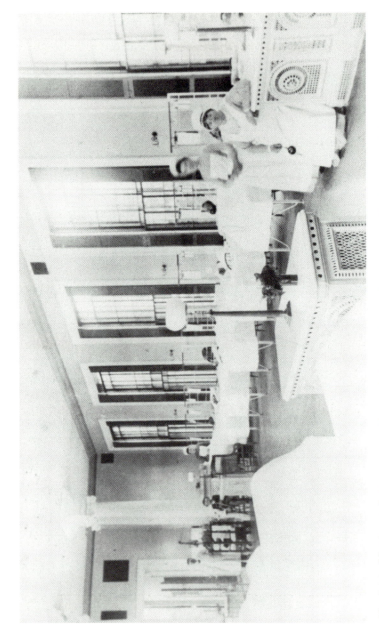

Fig. 3.36 Men's ward. Boston City Hospital, Boston, Massachusetts, c. 1885 (Countway Library).

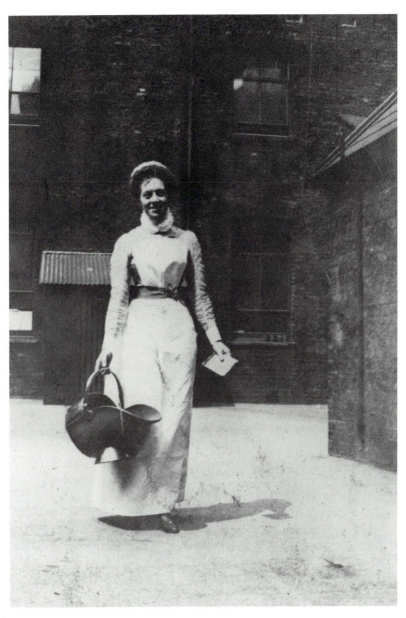

Fig. 3.37 St. Bartholomew's Hospital, London, a nurse, c. 1900. This was no doubt taken as a private portrait (Wellcome Institute Library, London).

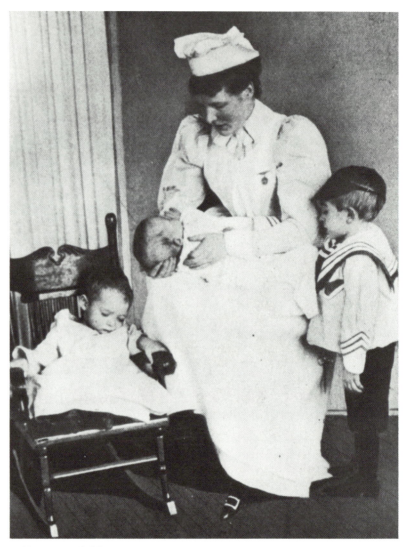

Fig. 3.38 Children's ward. Massachusetts Charitable Eye and Ear Infirmary, Boston, Massachusetts, 1898 (Jane Hodson, ed., *How to Become a Trained Nurse*, New York: A. Abbatt, 1898).

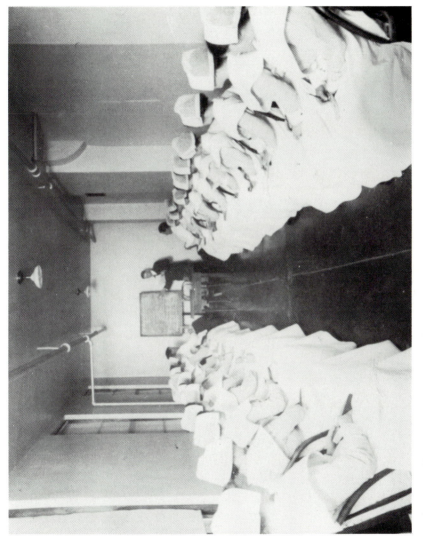

Fig. 3.39 Nurses' Lecture room, State Insane Hospital, Nebraska, 1914 (Nebraska Historical Society).

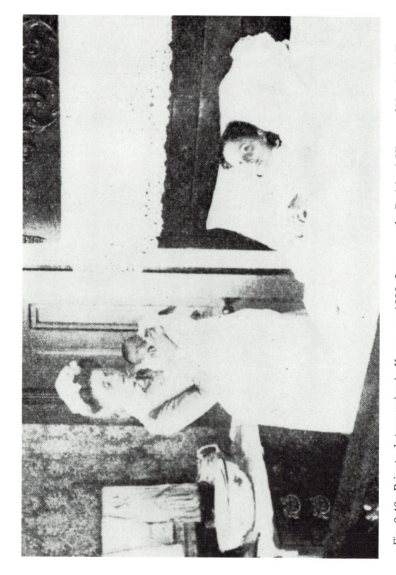

Fig. 3.40 Private duty nursing in Kansas. c. 1890. *Lamps on the Prairie: A History of Nursing in Kansas* (Topeka, Kansas: Kansas State Nurses' Association, 1942).

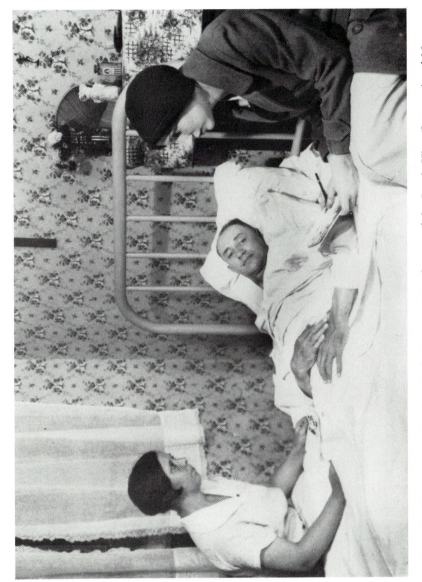

Fig. 3.41 Home nursing in New York City, c. 1915. Photograph by Lewis Hine (International Museum of Photography, Eastman House, Rochester, New York).

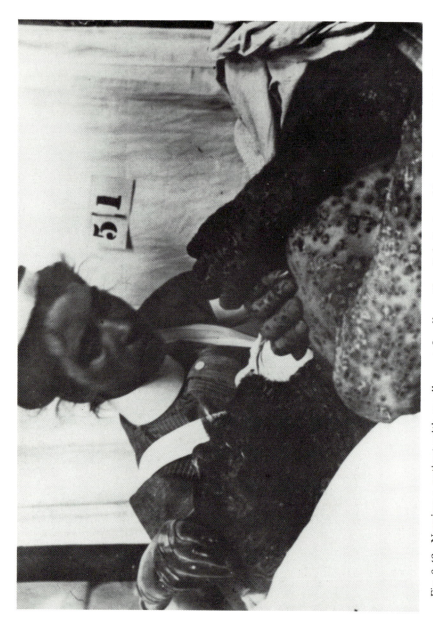

Fig. 3.42 Nursing a patient with smallpox at Smallpox Hospital, Boston, Massachusetts, 1902 (Countway Library).

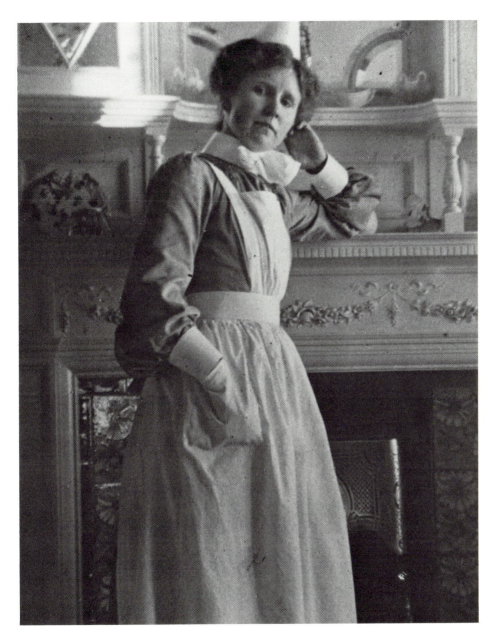

Fig. 3.43 Nurse at Montrose Asylum by W. C. Orkney, n.d. (Courtesy of the Angus Unit of the Tayside Health Board and Mr. Tom King, Medical Illustration Department of Dundee University).

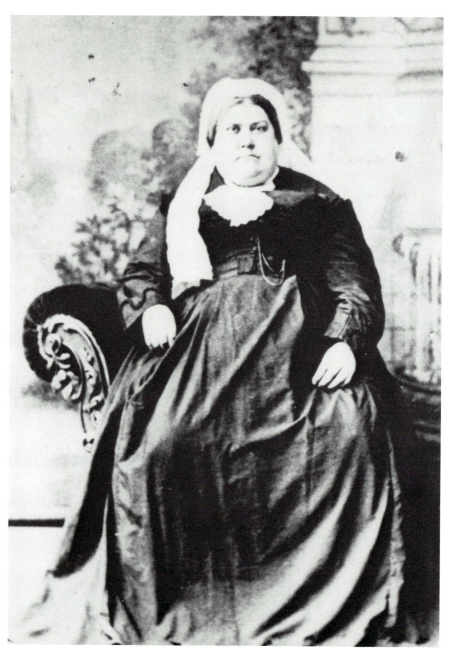

Fig. 3.44 Nurse at Leeds General Infirmary, 1873. This was a nurse who had not undergone any formal training (Leeds General Infirmary—17-625/1).

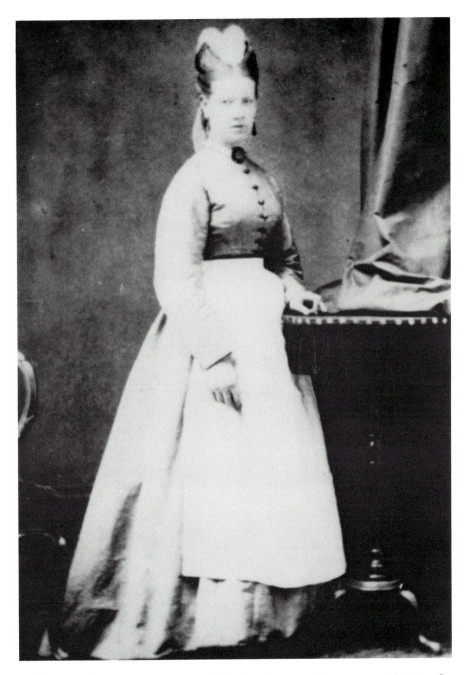

Fig. 3.45 A probationary nurse at Leeds General Infirmary, 1873. Nurses first began to be trained at Leeds when the new infirmary was opened in 1869 (Leeds General Infirmary—17-625/11).

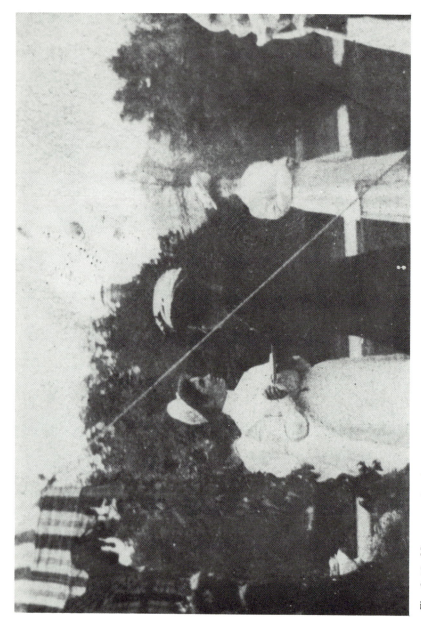

Fig. 3.46 Nurses and other women, Johns Hopkins Hospital, Baltimore, Maryland, c. 1910 (Alan Mason Chesney Archives of the Johns Hopkins University Medical Institutions).

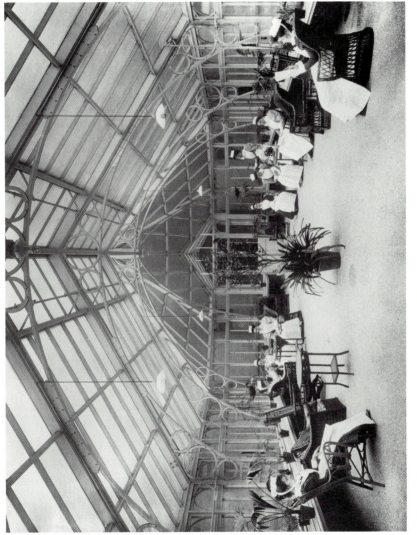

Fig. 3.47 Nurses' sitting room, Birmingham General Hospital, 1897. Conservatories were a regular feature of Victorian country houses (Birmingham General Hospital).

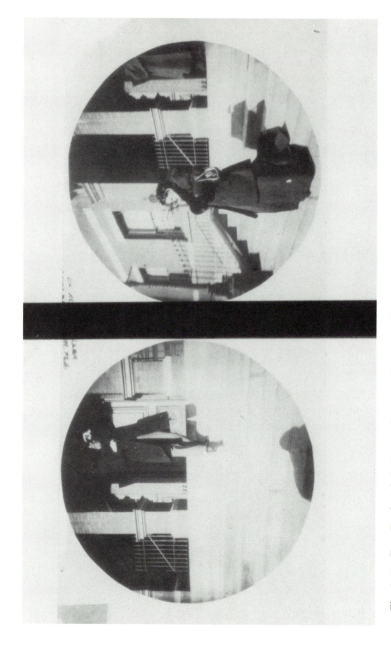

Fig. 3.48 Drs. Frederick P. Henry (left) and Eleanor C. Jones (right) on the steps of the hospital of what was then called Women's Medical College, 1898 (Archives and Special Collections on Women in Medicine, Medical College of Pennsylvania).

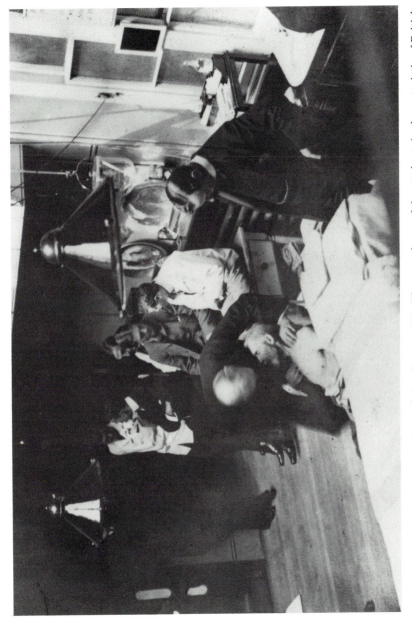

Fig. 3.49 St. Bartholomew's Hospital, London, c. 1900. The casualness of the students is characteristic of British photographs (Wellcome Institute Library, London).

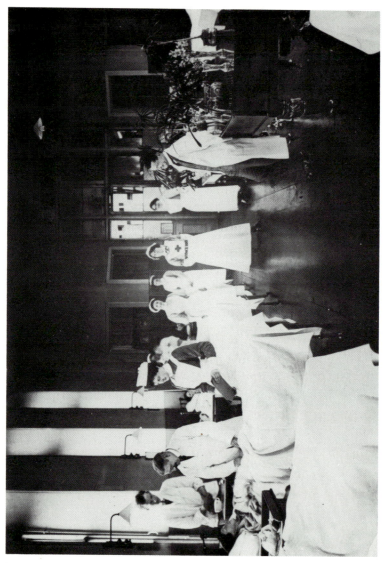

Fig. 3.50 A consultation on the wards of the Royal Infirmary, Edinburgh, c. 1905. Photographs of white coated senior physicians may have been less uncommon in Scotland, where the practice of medicine was regarded equally as a profession and as a gentlemanly vocation. In addition, this was a surgical ward (Royal Infirmary of Edinburgh—R10730/20).

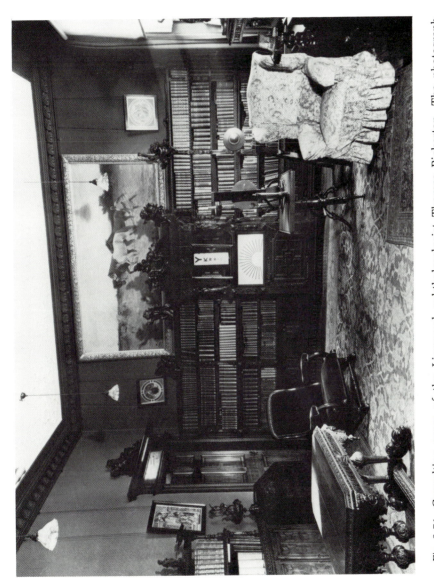

Fig. 3.51 Consulting room of the Liverpool ophthalmologist Thomas Bickerton. The photograph displays a genteel study while drawing attention to the eye-testing chart (Wellcome Institute Library, London).

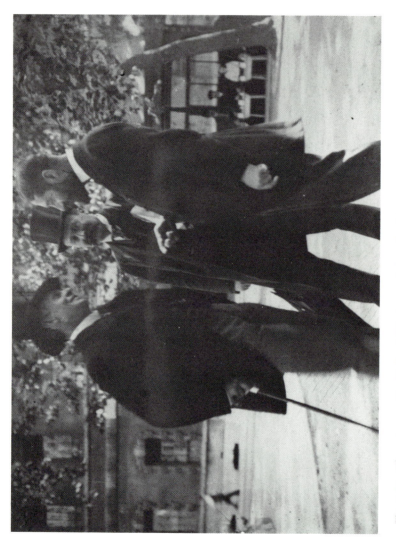

Fig. 3.52 The surgeon Sir Holbert Waring and the physicians J. Calvert and Wilmot Herringham converse in the grounds of St. Bartholomew's Hospital, London, c. 1900. See Geoffrey Bourne, *We Met at Bart's* (London: Frederick Muller, 1963) facing p. 113, for another such triad. Other examples of a similar configuration exist (Wellcome Institute Library, London).

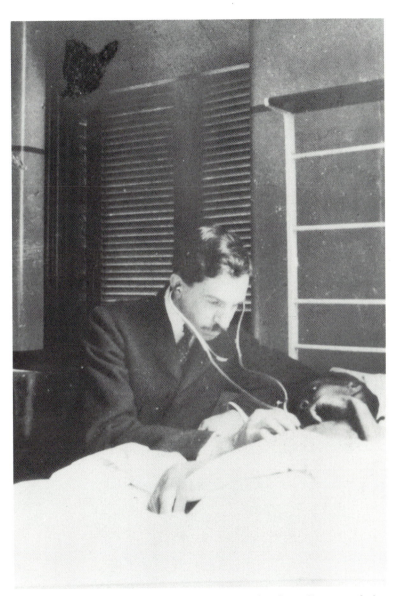

Fig. 3.53 Rufus Cole, who later became the first director of the hospital of the Rockefeller Institute for Medical Research in New York, is depicted in the 1890s, examining a child at the Johns Hopkins Hospital (Yale Medical Historical Library, New Haven, Connecticut).

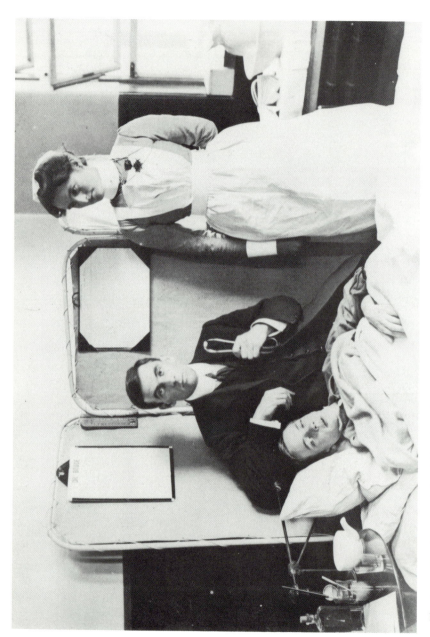

Fig. 3.54 The physician Basil Hood in the infectious diseases block, Charing Cross Hospital, London, 1904. This picture is quite unusual, both because it is a physician at the bedside and because of the prominence given to the stethoscope (Wellcome Institute Library, London).

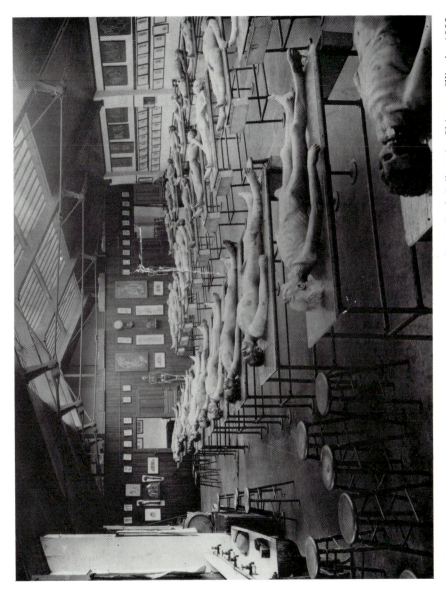

Fig. 3.55 Cadavers laid out in the dissecting room at Rush Medical College in Chicago, Illinois, 1900 (State Historical Society of Wisconsin, c. file 8).

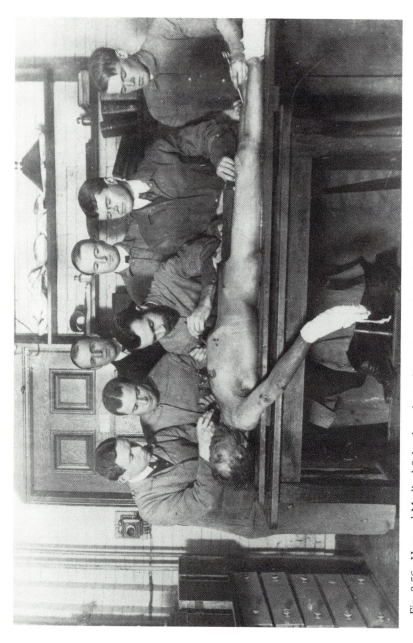

Fig. 3.56 Harvard Medical School students dissecting a cadaver in 1905. Many of these commemorative photographs depict the students clowning. Perhaps these students wanted to be represented as studious in the presence of a faculty member, the third person from the left (Countway Library).

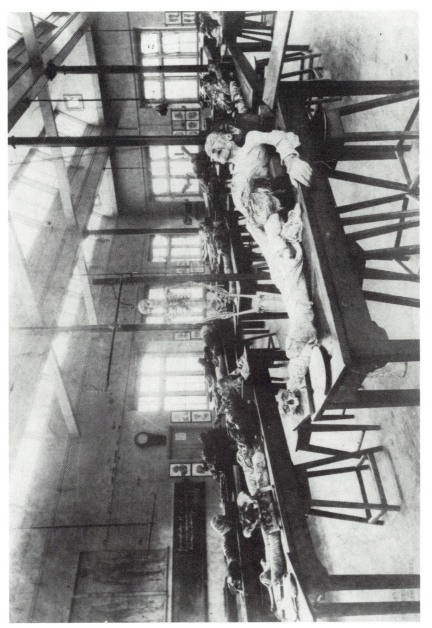

Fig. 3.57 Anatomy classroom at Cambridge University "by Stearn Cambridge," c. 1890 (Wellcome Institute Library, London).

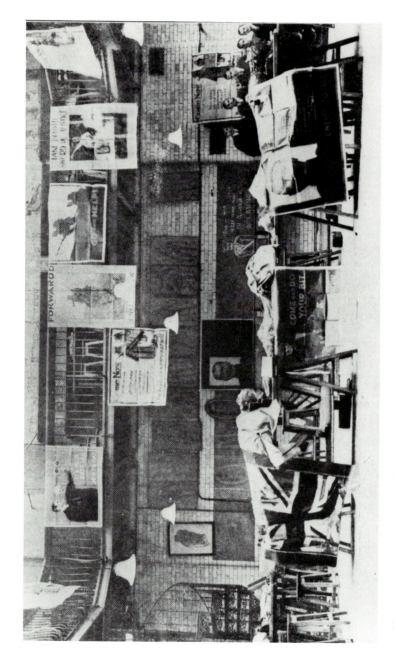

Fig. 3.58 Picture entitled "The dissecting rooms on 'Derby Day,' November 5th 1915," in Paul Bousfield, "Medical Students and the War," *St. Bartholomew's Hospital Journal 23* (1915):26-30 (Wellcome Institute Library, London).

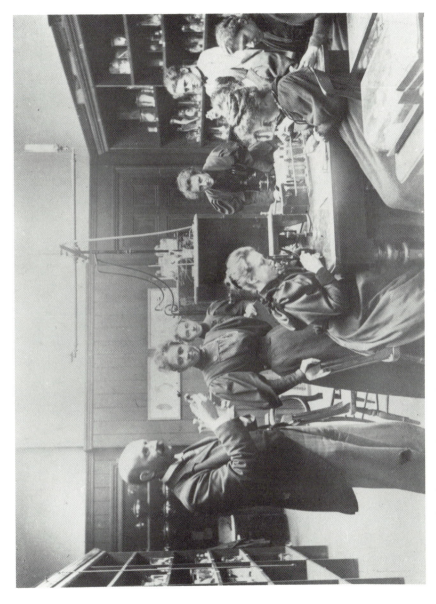

Fig. 3.59 The physician F. W. Andrews teaching in the pathology museum, Royal Free Hospital, c. 1890 (Royal Free Hospital School of Medicine).

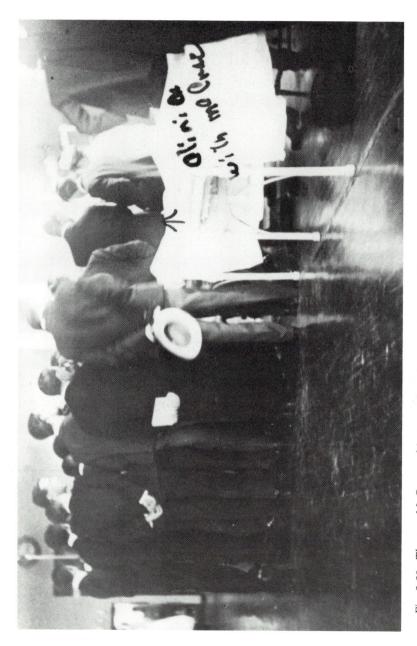

Fig. 3.60 Thomas McCrae making rounds at the Johns Hopkins Hospital, c. 1900. This photograph was included in a commemorative album put together by students (Alan Mason Chesney Medical Archives, the Johns Hopkins Medical Institution).

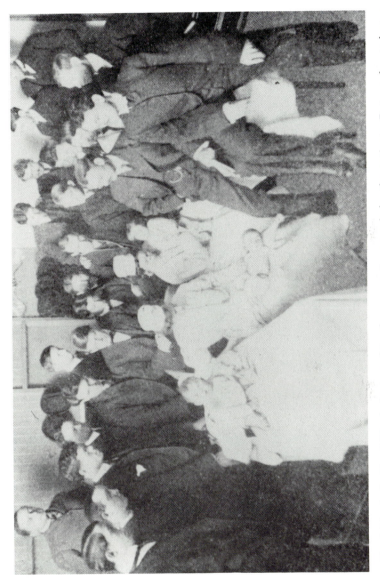

Fig. 3.61 As in Fig. 3.60, students and teachers seem to overwhelm the patients. But we do not know how these pictures were perceived at the turn of the century. This photograph depicts a class in clinical pediatrics at the Northwestern University College of Medicine in Chicago, in 1906 (*The Neoplasm*, Northwestern University College of Medicine, Yearbook, 1906. Northwestern University Medical School Archives).

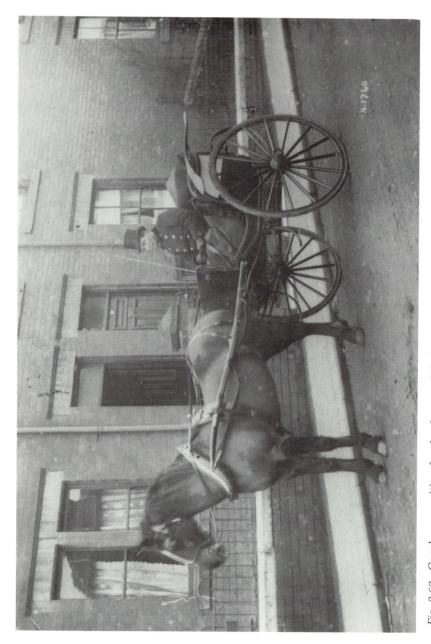

Fig. 3.62 Coachman waiting for the doctor while he makes a house call in Stanley, County Durham, c. 1910. A remarkable number of photographs rather like this exist (Beamish North of England Open Air Museum, Durham— 84 65).

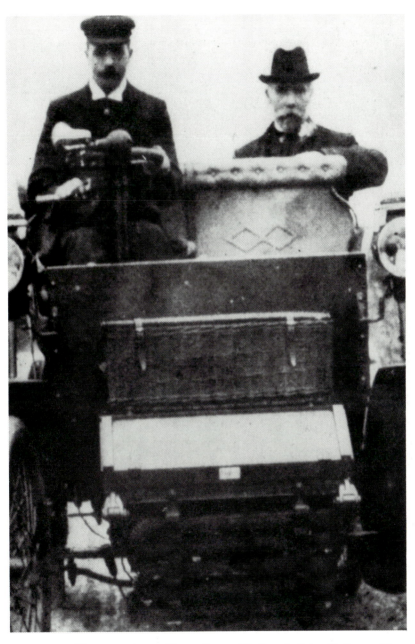

Fig. 3.63 The general practitioner James Mackenzie (later Sir James Mac-kenzie) on his rounds in Burnley with his chauffeur, c. 1900 (*Canadian Medical Association Journal*, 1962, 87:551).

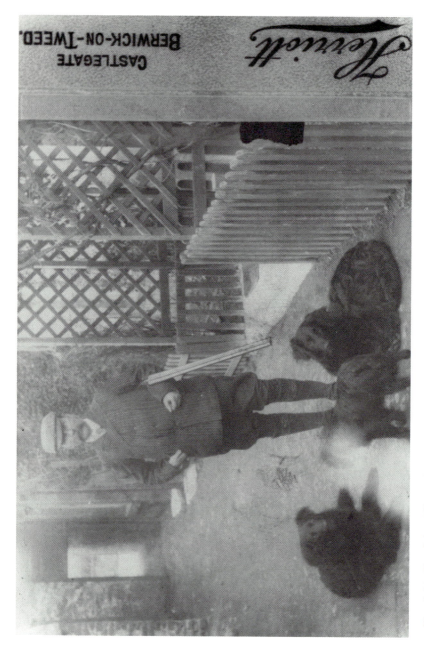

Fig. 3.64 Dr. John Elliot of Lowick, Northumberland, England, c. 1900 (Beamish North of England Open Air Museum, Durham—18199).

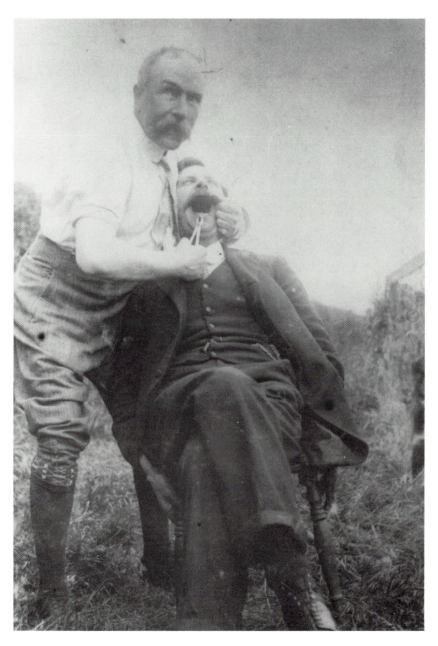

Fig. 3.65 Dr. John Elliot pulling teeth, c. 1900 (Beamish North of England Open Air Museum, Durham—18197).

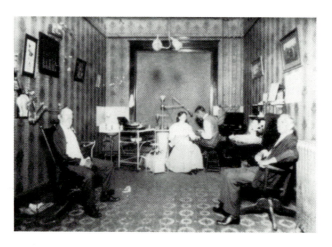

Fig. 3.66 A doctor's office and waiting room in Wichita, Kansas, c. 1895 (Medical Society of Sedgwick County, Kansas).

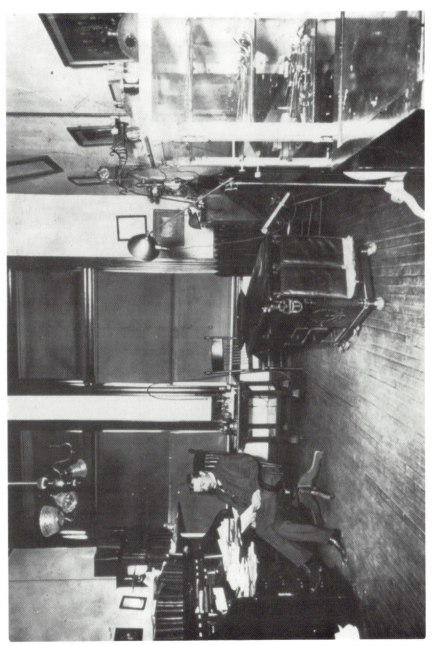

Fig. 3.67 A doctor in his office in Minneapolis, Minnesota, c. 1900. The shades were drawn to exclude glare during photography (Minnesota Historical Society, Special Libraries).

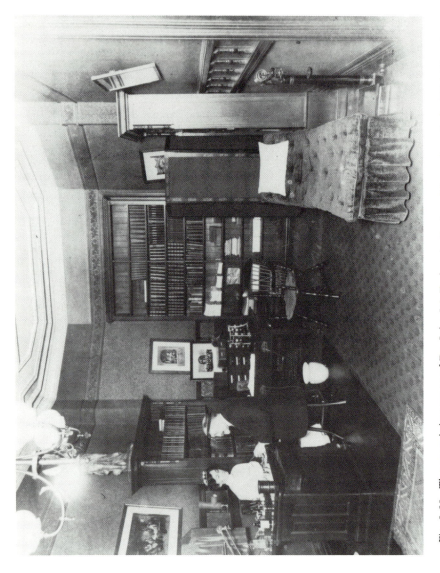

Fig. 3.68 The examining room of Dr. John W. Farlow in Boston, Massachusetts in 1914 (Countway Library).

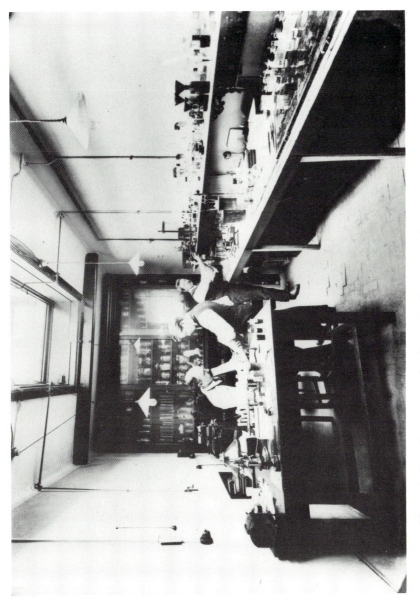

Fig. 3.69 The pathology department, the Great Northern Central Hospital, London, 1912. This pathologist was represented taking blood from a patient, with a laboratory bench on the right and a pathology museum in the background. St. Bartholomew's produced a postcard of its pathology laboratory at this time (Wellcome Institute Library, London).

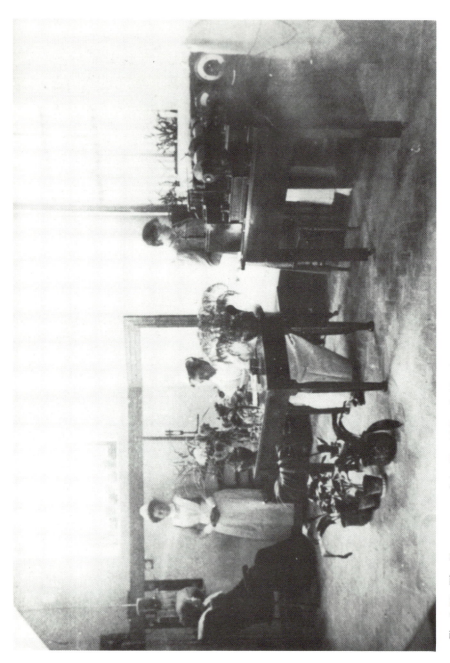

Fig. 3.70 The X-ray room of the David Lewis Northern Hospital, Liverpool, 1902. Note the nurses in their conventional ward postures (Courtesy of Dr. T. Cook).

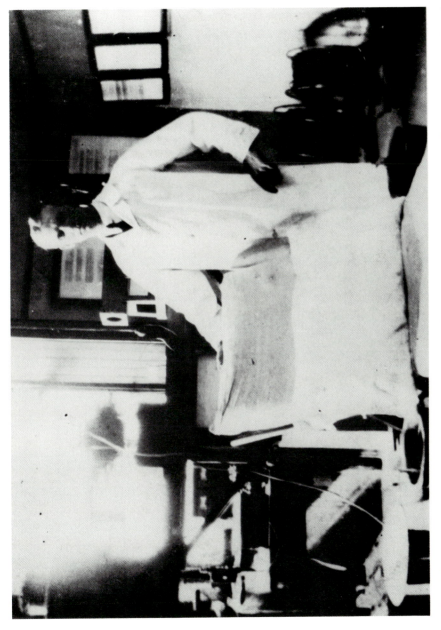

Fig. 3.71 The first electrocardiograph and a technician in the Royal Infirmary of Edinburgh, 1911 (Royal Infirmary of Edinburgh—R10730/8).

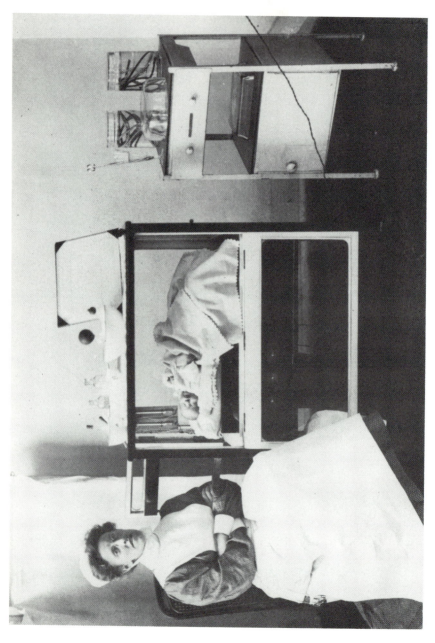

Fig. 3.72 Nurse with incubator 1908. From the album of Dr. Basil Hood, Charing Cross Hospital. Incubators were invented at the end of the nineteenth century, and were a very popular photographic subject (Wellcome Institute Library, London).

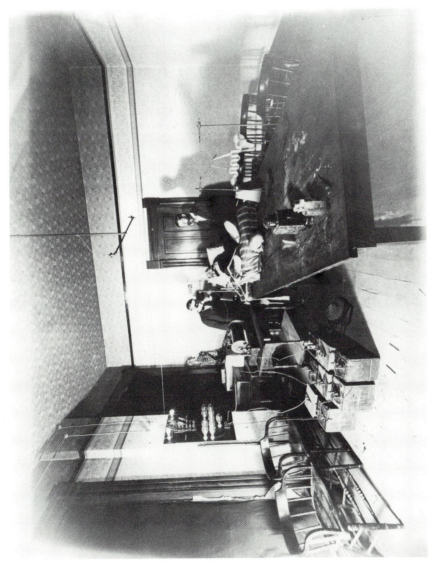

Fig. 3.73 This photograph, taken at St. Luke's Hospital in Denver, Colorado, in 1896, is said to depict the first X-ray of a patient in the state (Amon Carter Museum, Fort Worth, Texas—Mazulla Collection).

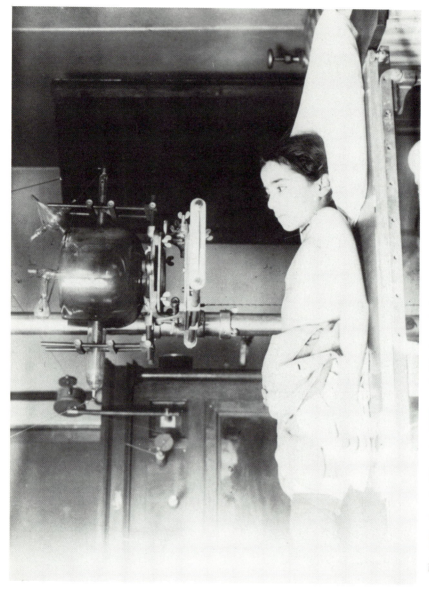

Fig. 3.74 Lewis Hine, in 1915, probably intended viewers to make a contrast between the patient and technology (International Museum of Photography, Eastman House, Rochester, New York).

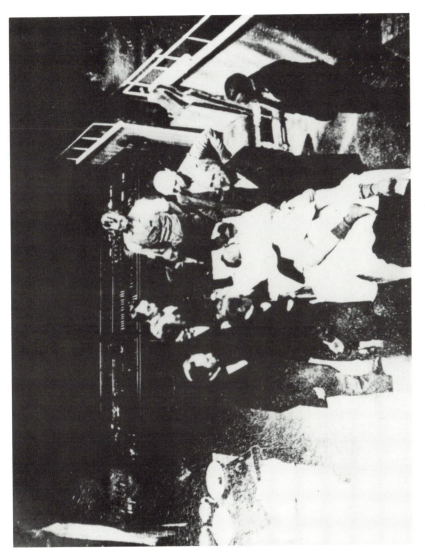

Fig. 3.75 This photograph of an early operation under ether, taken at the Massachusetts General Hospital in 1846 by Josiah J. Hawes, has probably been published more often than any other image of American medicine. Even if it was simulated, it is a typical representation of surgery in the mid-nineteenth century (Library of Congress, Manuscript Division, Helman Collection).

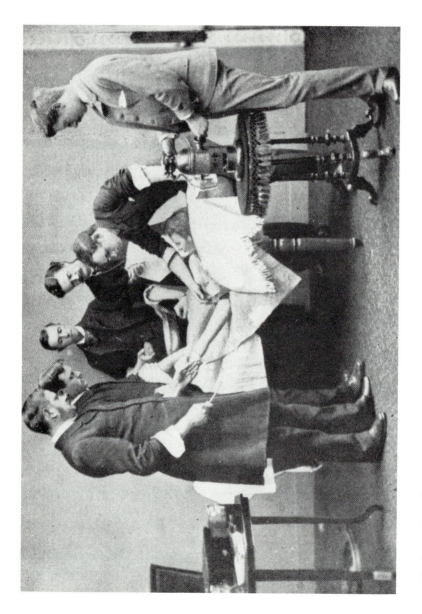

Fig. 3.76 Described as an operation at Aberdeen, c. 1880. This may also have been a simulation. This picture was composed to make the Lister spray prominent. Surgical pictures from this date often show the surgeon poised, knife in hand. See D. Guthrie, *Lord Lister: His Life and Doctrine* (Edinburgh: Livingstone, 1949) (Courtesy of Churchill Livingstone, original untraceable).

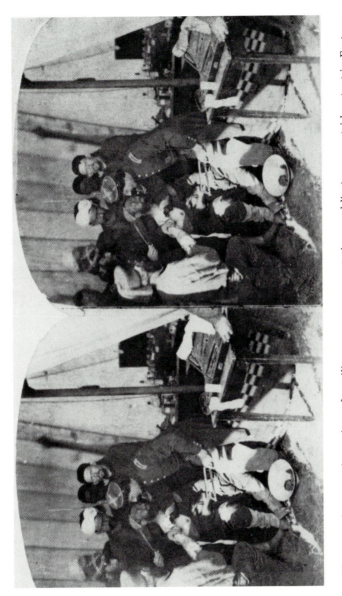

Fig. 3.77 A stereopticon view of a military surgeon amputating a soldier's arm outside a tent in Fortress Monroe, Virginia, c. 1863 (Edward G. Miner Library, University of Rochester School of Medicine and Dentistry).

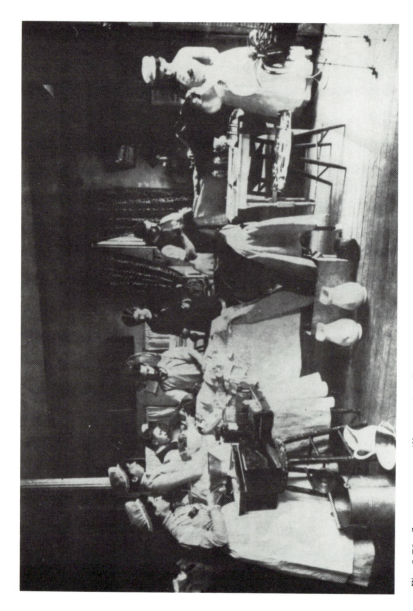

Fig. 3.78 Surgery was still occasionally represented as a public activity, even in the 1880s. This photograph depicts an operation on a ward at Bellevue Hospital in the late 1880s (National Library of Medicine).

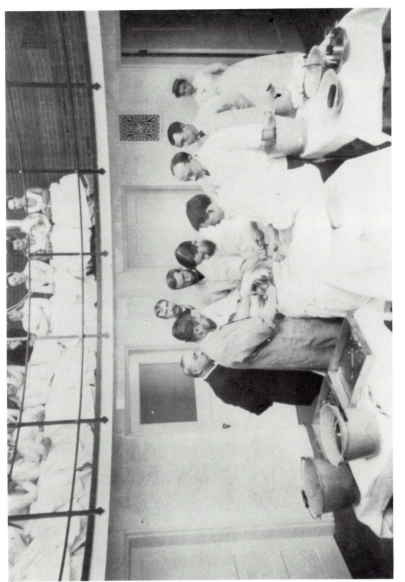

Fig. 3.79　Abdominal ward amphitheater, Massachusetts General Hospital, 1888 (Countway Library).

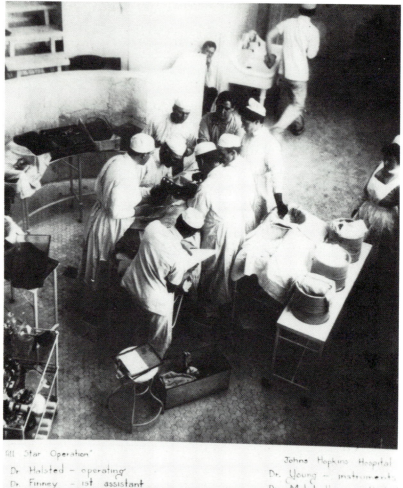

"All Star Operation"

Johns Hopkins Hospital

Dr. Halsted – operating
Dr. Finney – 1st assistant
Dr. Cushing – 2nd assistant
Dr. Bloodgood – 3rd assistant

Dr. Young – instruments
Dr. Mitchell – anaesthetist
Dr. Follis – leaving
Dr. Baetjer – seated

Miss Hampton – operating nurse

Fig. 3.80 This photograph was signed and called "The All-Star Operation." The departing figure at the upper right is the only person not identified in the original caption. He may be the man in the right foreground in the photograph (Fig. 1.3), which was not used as a souvenir of the occasion (Yale Medical Historical Library).

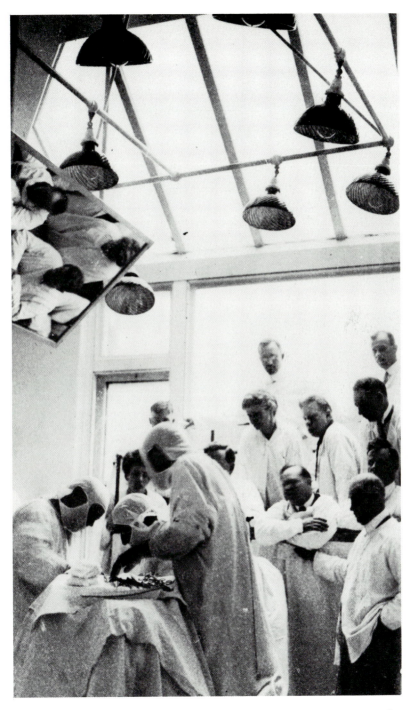

Fig. 3.81 Charles H. Mayo, in the left foreground, operating at St. Mary's Hospital, Rochester, Minnesota, 1911 (Mayo Clinic—01164).

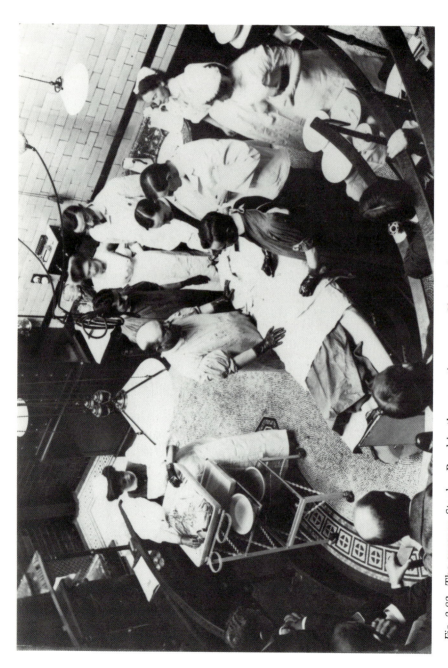

Fig. 3.82 The surgeon Stanley Boyd in the operating room, Charing Cross Hospital London, 1900. From the Basil Hood Album. This is possibly the first overhead photograph of a surgical operation in Britain (Wellcome Institute Library, London).

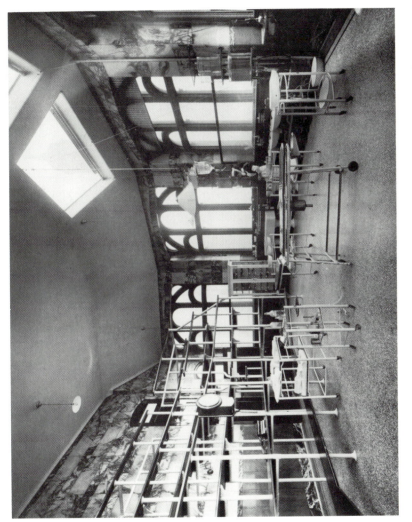

Fig. 3.83 The operating theatre of the newly opened General Hospital, Birmingham, 1897. From a commemorative album. Such pictures are quite common after this time. The nurse poses in the usual manner, but the theatre is represented as somewhere quite different from a domestic area (Birmingham General Hospital).

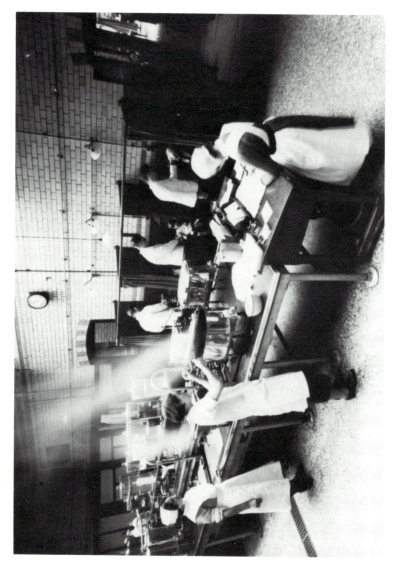

Fig. 3.84 The accident department, University College Hospital, c. 1910. Central to this image of medicine at work is the preparation for surgery. The nurse on the left stands in the conventional way, but the other two women are working (The Library, University College Hospital, London).

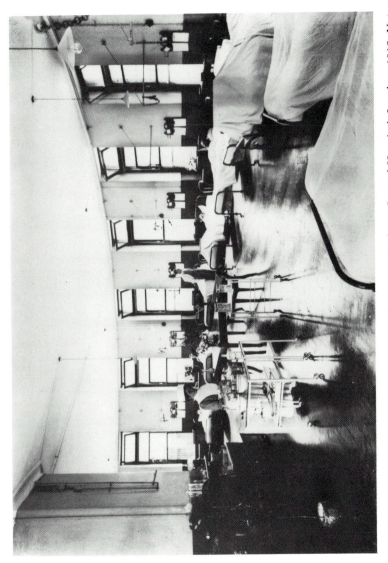

Fig. 3.85 Picture of Cloudesley Ward at the Great Northern Central Hospital, London, 1912. Note the prominence of the surgical dressing trolleys. Four of the ward pictures in the album containing this photograph have dressing trolleys in the foreground. See also Fig. 0.2 (Wellcome Institute Library, London).

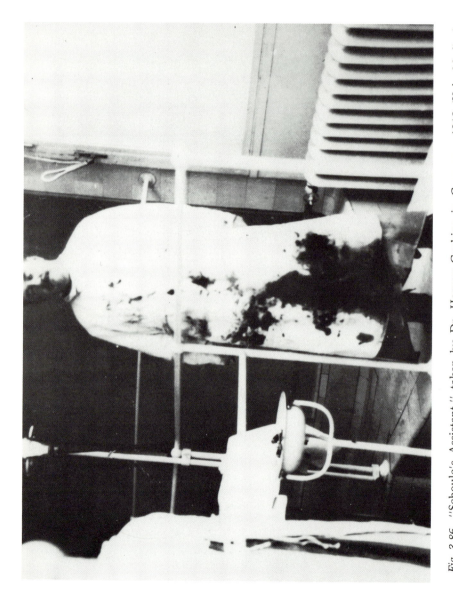

Fig. 3.86 "Schoule's Assistant," taken by Dr. Harvey Cushing in Germany, 1912 (Yale Medical Historical Library).

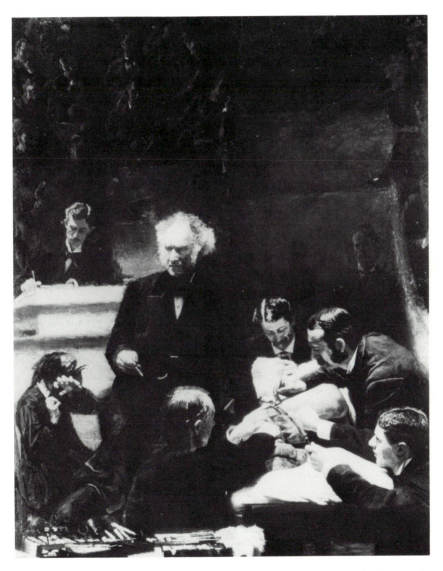

Fig. 3.87 Samuel Gross of Philadelphia presiding over his surgical clinic. Oil painting by Thomas Eakins, 1875 (Thomas Jefferson University).

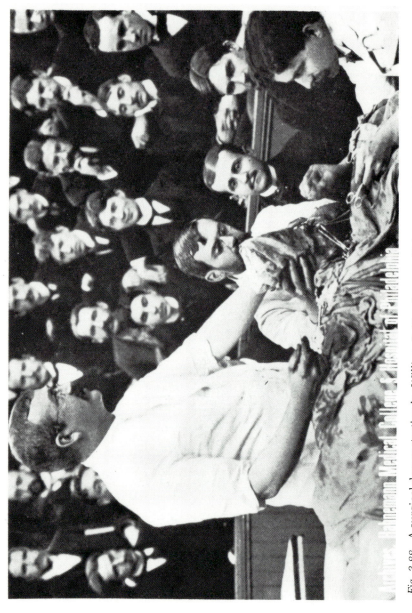

Fig. 3.88 A surgical demonstration by William B. Van Lennep, Hahnemann Hospital, Philadelphia, Pennsylvania, 1899 (Hahnemann University Archives and Medical History Collections. Hahnemann Class Book).

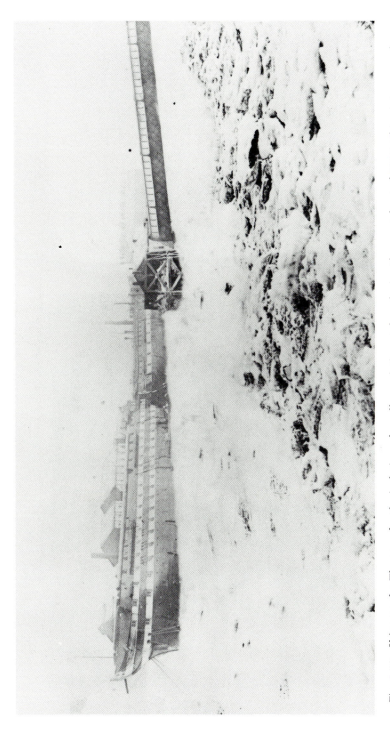

Fig. 3.89 Ships on the Thames, for the isolation of smallpox victims, taken during the great frost of 1890. This picture may have been taken for aesthetic purposes. Since the photograph is in the collection of Greater London Photograph Library, this seems unlikely, as the collection contains a large number of pictures from around the same time chronicling medical activities. Smallpox hospital photographs are not rare, and usually depict something temporary and isolated, tents in a field for example (By courtesy of Greater London Photograph Library—84/425).

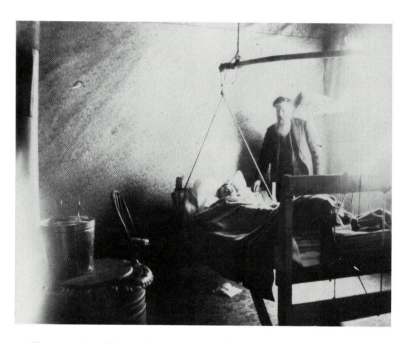

Fig. 3.90 A public isolation hospital, or pest house, in Idaho, c. 1890. The patient has typhoid fever; the rope and pulley may have been used to lift the patient for bathing (Idaho Historical Society).

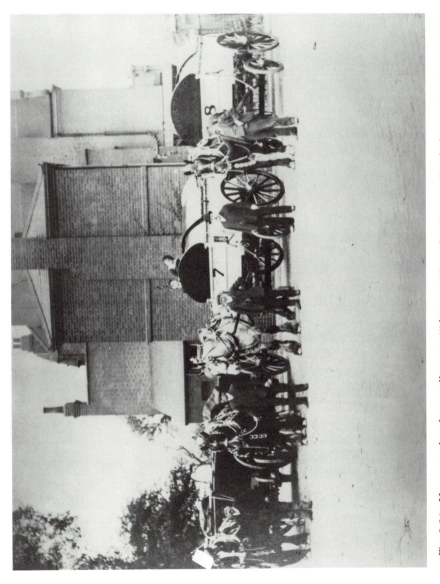

Fig. 3.91 Hampstead refuse collectors ("dustmen") at Lymington Road depot, London, c. 1905 (London Borough of Camden Local History Library—80/1153).

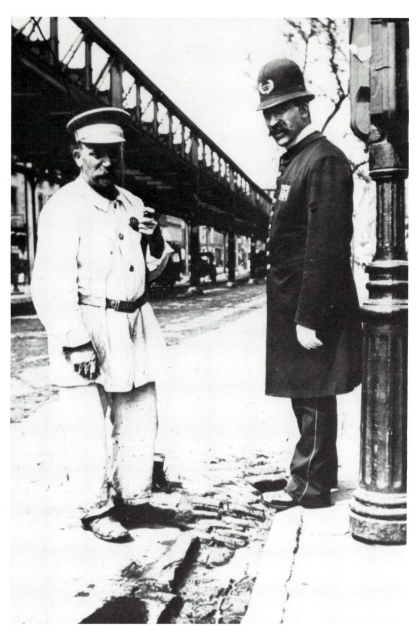

Fig. 3.92 A policeman and a health inspector in New York City, May 9, 1896. The noted photographer, Alice Austin, probably did not set out to depict public health practice as a policing function of government (Staten Island Historical Society—E-235).

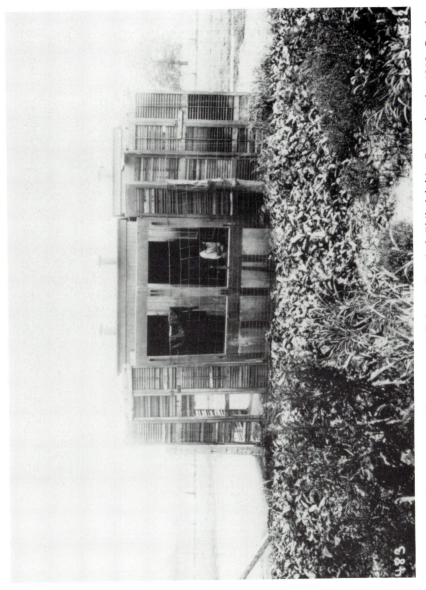

Fig. 3.93 Outhouses, one with a person, at Byberry Hospital, Philadelphia, Pennsylvania, 1912. Caption reads "toilet for the depressed" (Philadelphia City Archives).

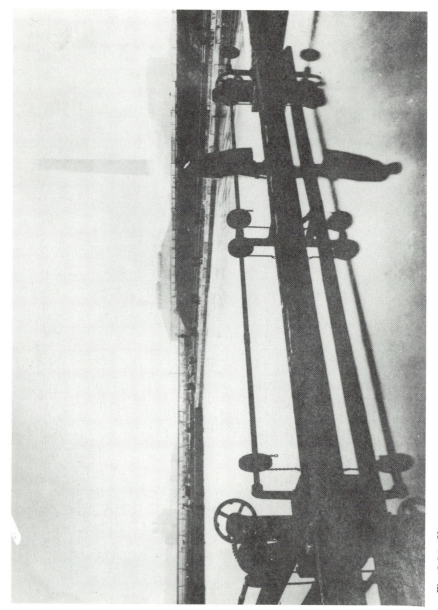

Fig. 3.94 Knostrop sewage works, Leeds, England, c. 1910 (Leeds City Libraries).

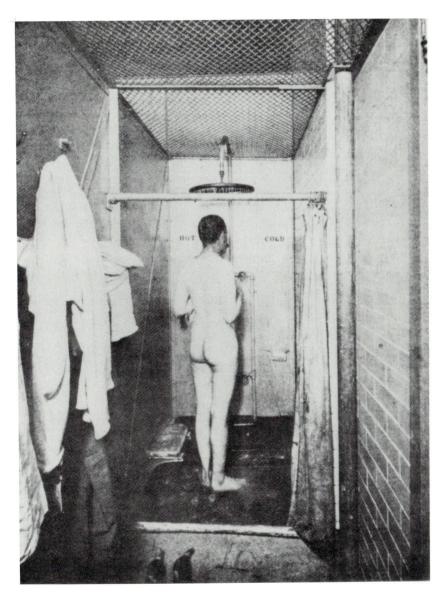

Fig. 3.95 A philanthropic public bath, New York, c. 1900. R. W. De Forest, L. Veiller, *The Tenement House Problem* (New York: Macmillan, 1903).

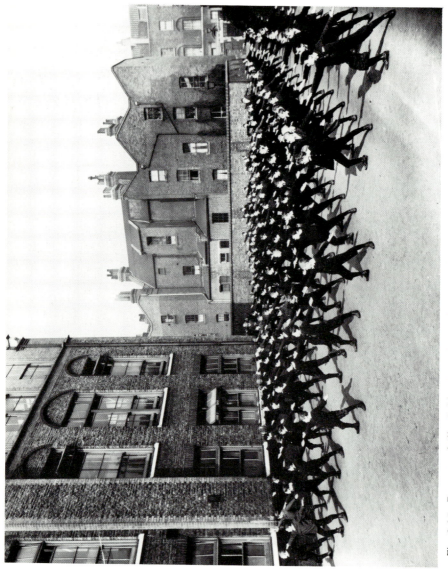

Fig. 3.96 Boys at drill, Cable St. School, London, 1908 (Greater London Photograph Library— 66/7751).

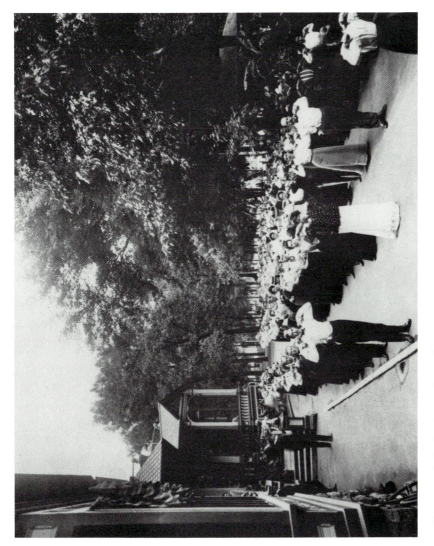

Fig. 3.97 Calisthenics at the Kellog Sanitarium, Battle Creek, Michigan, around 1900 (Michigan Historical Collections [UA2], University of Michigan).

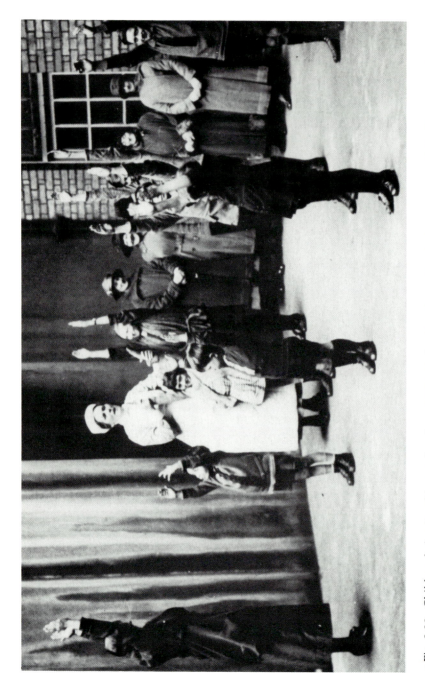

Fig. 3.98 Children being taught exercises by a nurse at the Middlesex Hospital, London, c. 1910. This hospital nurse, unusually, is represented as actively engaged in a task. However, this was the normal representation of women involved in public health work (The Archivist of the Middlesex Hospital).

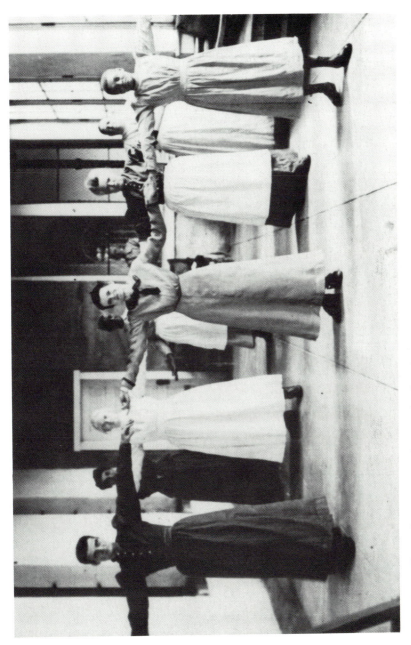

Fig. 3.99 Physical exercise as therapy for female patients in the "violent ward" of Columbus State Hospital in Ohio, c. 1911 (Ohio Historical Society).

153

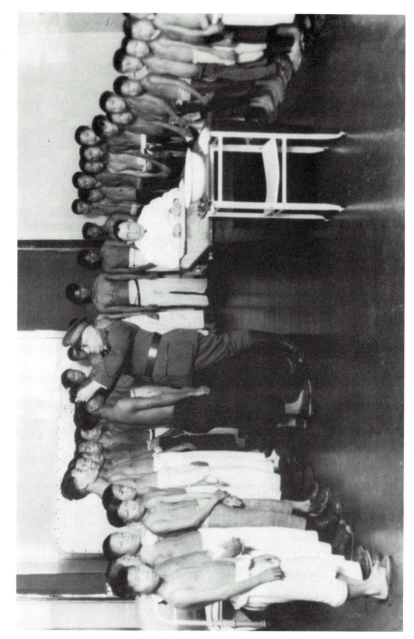

Fig. 3.100 Health inspection of immigrants from Asia, Angel Island, California, c. 1900-1910 (National Archives of the United States).

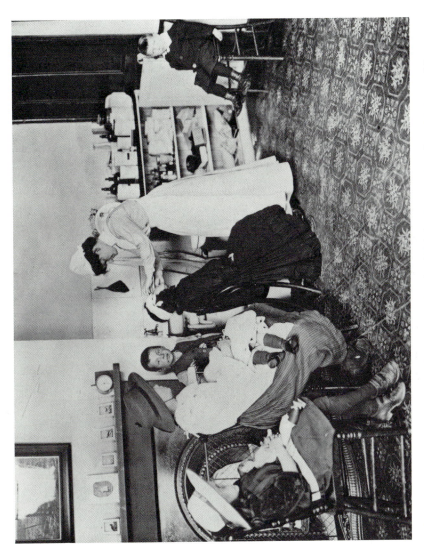

Fig. 3.101 A minor ailments clinic at the Deptford Health Centre, London, 1911. Health centres were local borough ventures providing public health services for the poor (Greater London Photograph Library—80/5357).

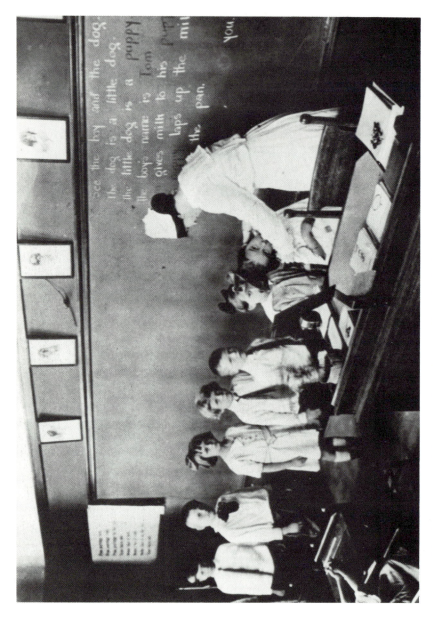

Fig. 3.102 A nurse examining school children in New York City, c. 1905. These inspections were usually performed by private physicians who were paid by the city's health department (National Library of Medicine).

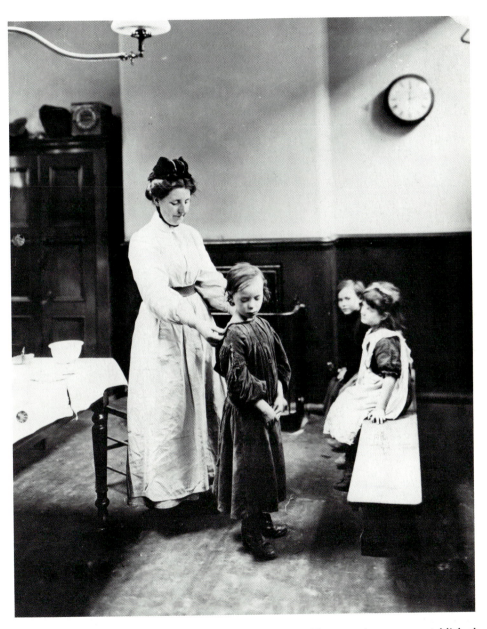

Fig. 3.103 Chaucer Cleansing station, London, 1911. These stations were established under an act of Parliament for the disinfecting and cleansing of verminous persons (By courtesy of Greater London Photograph Library—80/5350).

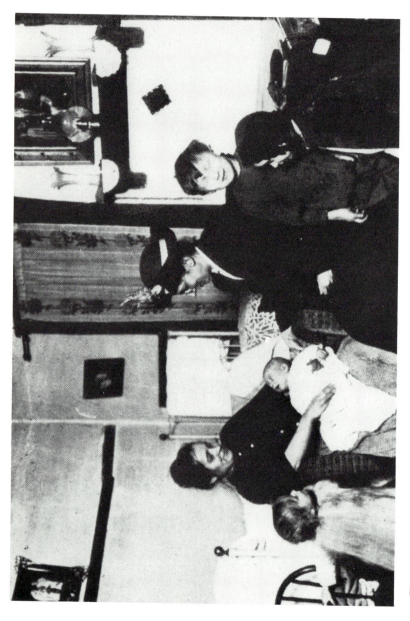

Fig. 3.104 A Lewis Hine photograph of a visiting nurse with a mother and three children in Homestead, Pennsylvania, a town built and owned by the Carnegie Steel Company, c. 1910. Paul U. Kellogg, *The Pittsburgh Survey: Findings in Six Volumes* (New York: Survey Associates for the Russell Sage Foundation, 1914).

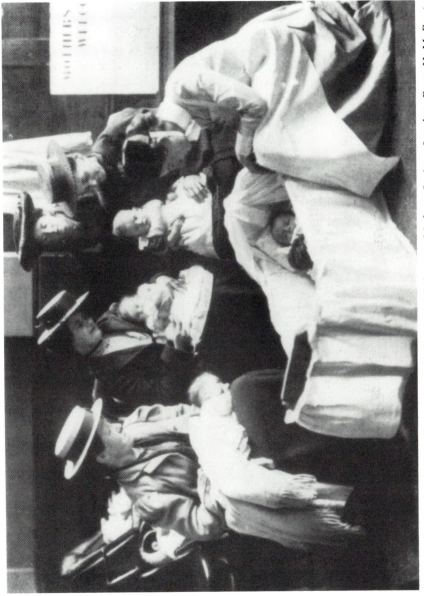

Fig. 3.105 Mothercraft being taught at St. Pancras, Mothers and Infants Society, London. From H. M. Bunting, et al., *A School for Mothers* (London: H. Marshall, 1907), frontispiece (Wellcome Institute Library, London).

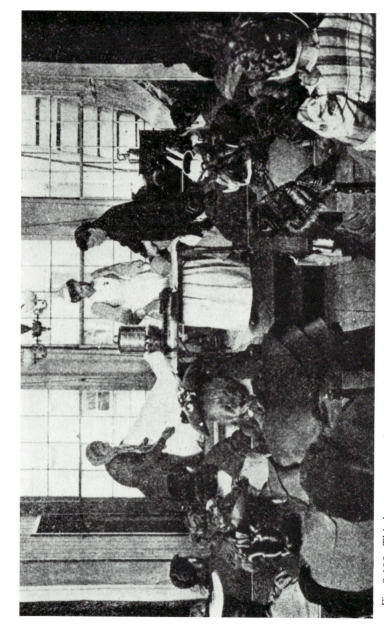

Fig. 3.106 This lesson was conducted at the Henry Street Settlement in New York City in 1906 (*Charities*, 1906, 16:34).

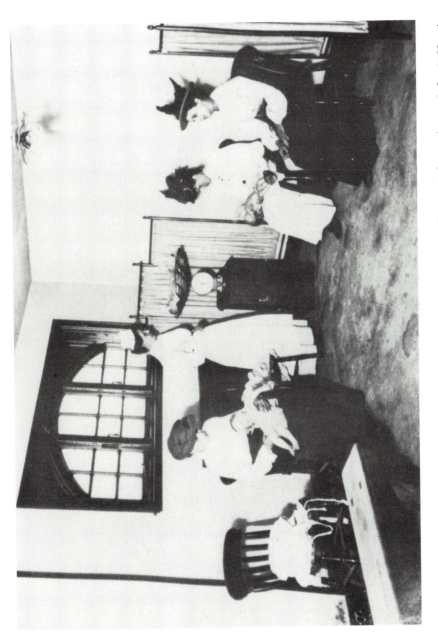

Fig. 3.107 The scale is the focal point of this photograph of a nurse weighing an infant, taken at Infant's Hospital, Westminster, c. 1908 [John Topham Picture Library, Kent].

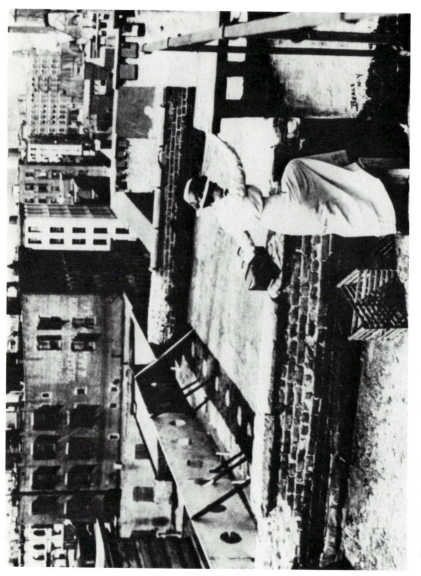

Fig. 3.108 A visiting nurse in New York City in 1910 taking a short-cut across the roof of a tenement. This is probably the most frequently reproduced photograph of home health care in the United States (Visiting Nurse Service of New York).

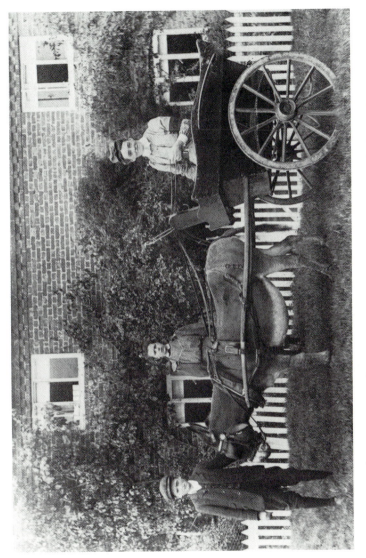

Fig. 3.109 A Queen's "Jubilee" nurse with her donkey cart at Gotheringham, Gloucestershire, c. 1895. Pictures of British nurses outside institutions are rare. Queen's nurses were district nurses, paid for from a fund raised by women in England in the year of Victoria's Jubilee, 1887. They did bedside nursing as well as teaching elementary hygiene. This picture was presumably taken to celebrate medical service to a rural community (Gloucestershire Records Office—D4057/26, courtesy Miss G. E. Brownhill).

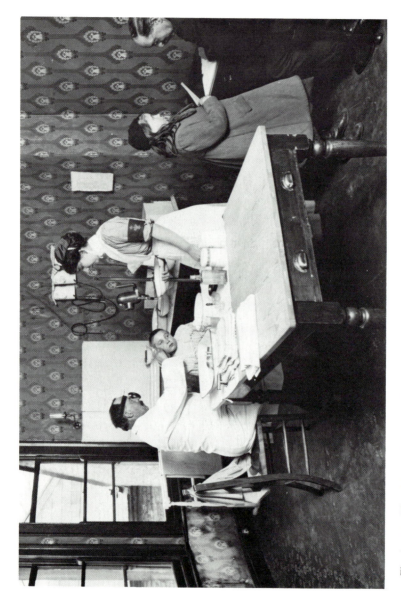

Fig. 3.110 The 'Minor Ailments Room,' Medical Treatment Centre Woolwich, London, 1914. This man and the one in the following picture were public employees who would also have had their own private practices. Examination is public, aggressive and uses surgical imagery (By courtesy of Greater London Photograph Library—80/5352).

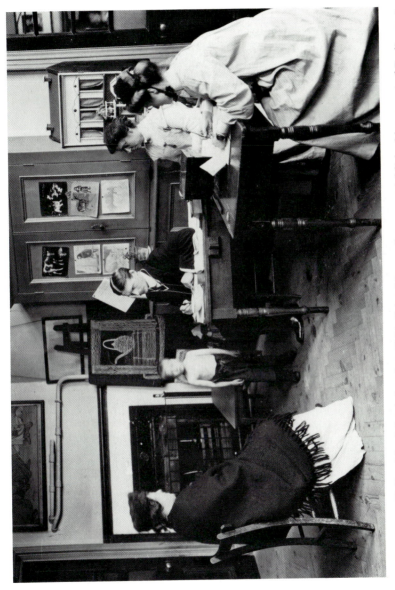

Fig. 3.111 Holland St. School, London 1911. School inspection was established by an act of Parliament of 1907. Once again, this is active medical work, among the poor (Greater London Photograph Library—70/3695).

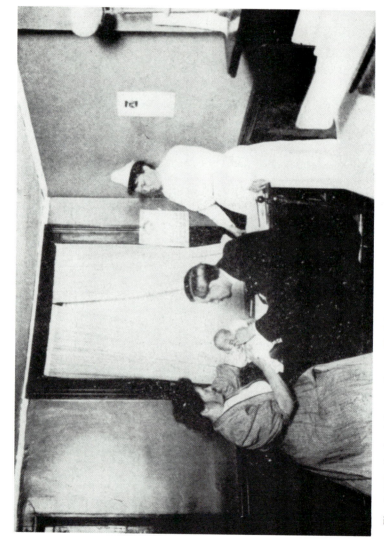

Fig. 3.112 A physician on the staff of the New York Milk Commission examining a child, c. 1910 (Social Welfare History Archives Center, University of Minnesota).

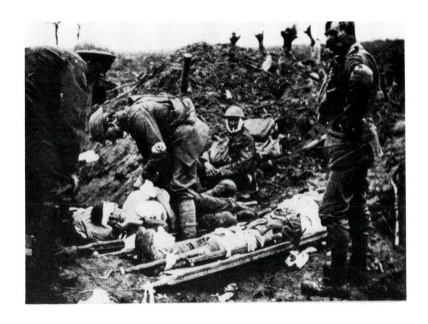

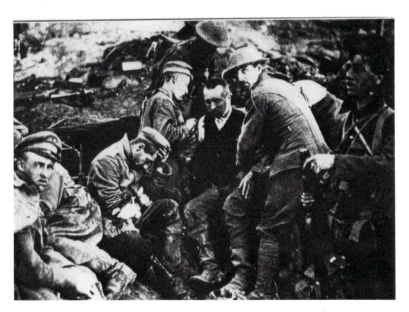

Fig. 3.113 Canadian Red Cross personnel treating wounded in Flanders, 1915. Top: dressing an officer's wounds on the battlefield. Below: attending wounded Germans at an advance dressing station. Woods Hutchinson, *The Doctor in War* (Boston: Houghton, Mifflin Co., 1918).

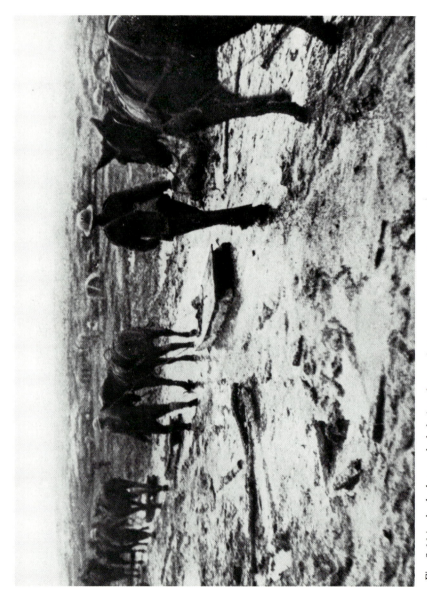

Fig. 3.114 Ambulance sleds being dragged through the mud, France, 1914-1918. Woods Hutchinson, *The Doctor in War* (Boston: Houghton, Mifflin Co., 1918).

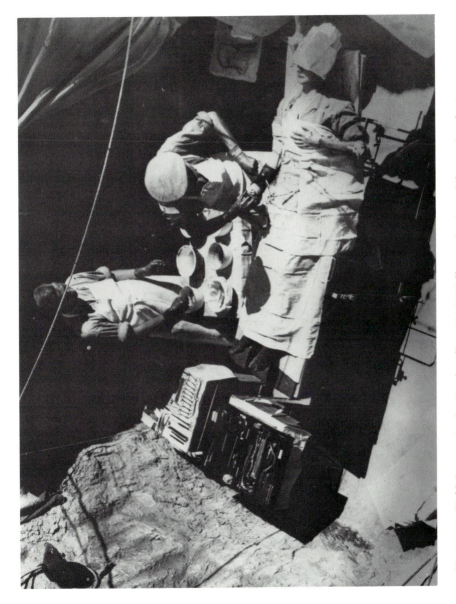

Fig. 3.115 Field Surgery in the Dardanelles, 1915 (Wellcome Institute Library, London).

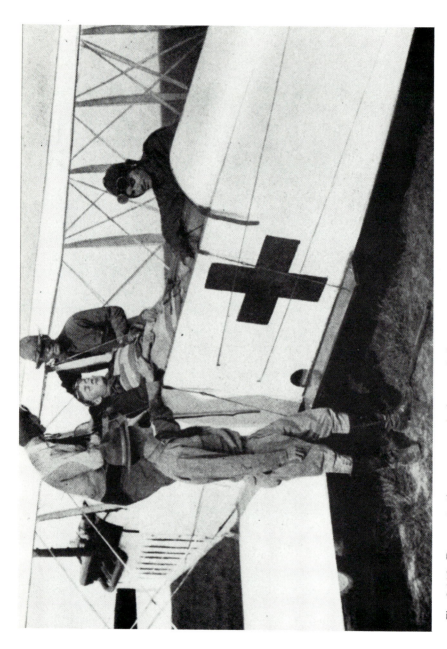

Fig. 3.116 Demonstrating an army airplane ambulance, c. 1918. From Edgar Erskine Hume, *Victories of Army Medicine; Scientific Accomplishments of the Medical Department of the United Stated Army* (Philadelphia: Lippincott, 1943, courtesy Alice J. Hume).

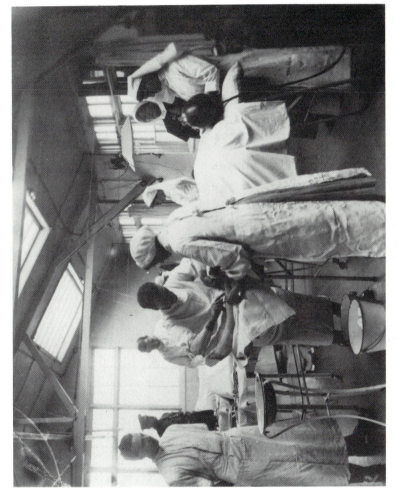

Fig. 3.117 Operating Theatre, Wimereux, World War I.

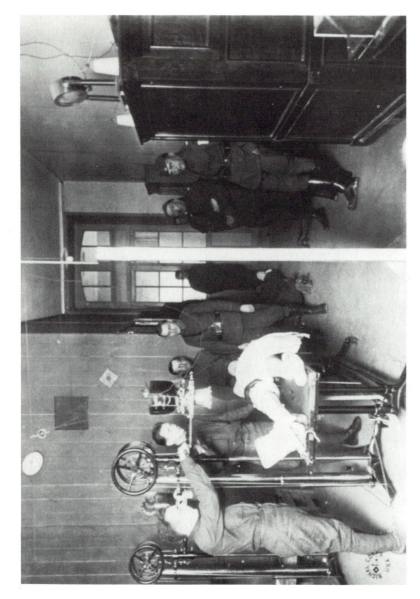

Fig. 3.118 X-raying a wounded man, United States Army Base Hospital, Savenay, France, 1918 (National Library of Medicine, United States Signal Corps).

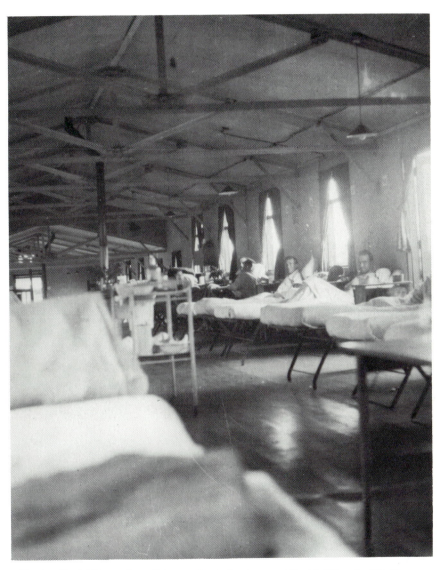

Fig. 3.119 Military hospital ward at Boulogne, World War I (Wellcome Institute Library, London).

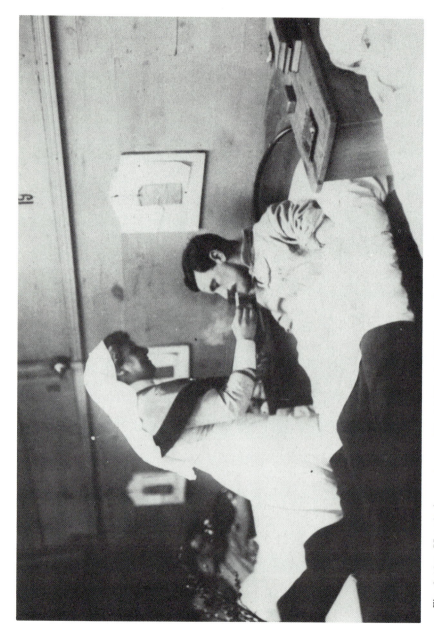

Fig. 3.120 Hospital on a barge, World War I (Wellcome Institute Library, London).

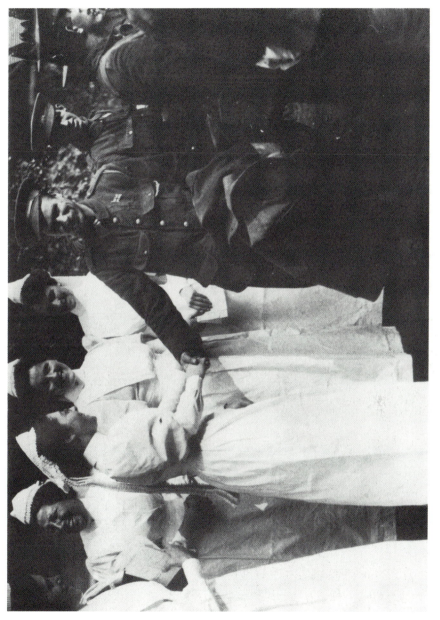

Fig. 3.121 London hospital nurses bidding goodbye to convalescent soldiers, World War I (Wellcome Institute Library, London).

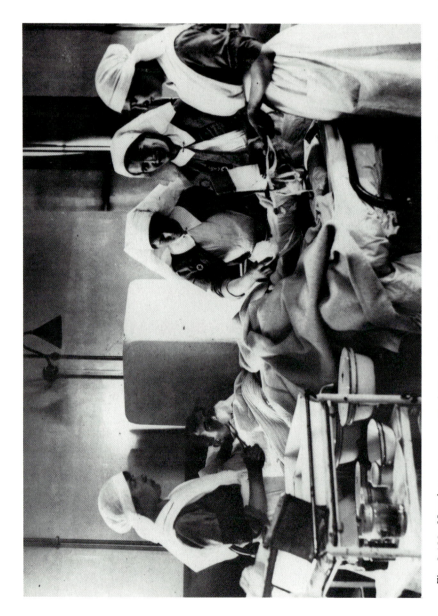

Fig. 3.122 Naval nurses on a Red Cross train at Chatham, with the heroes of Zeebrugge (Wellcome Institute Library, London).

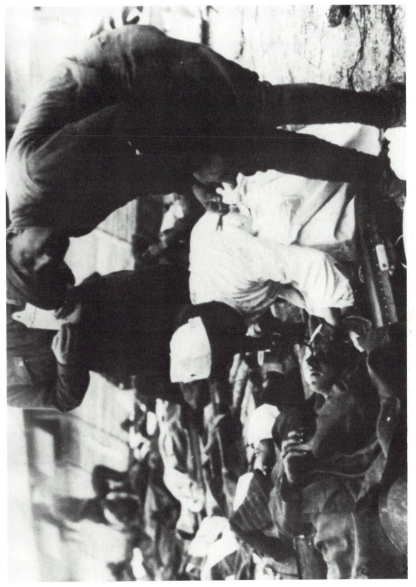

Fig. 3.123 After a gas attack, Field Hospital No. 326, Royamieux, France, 1918 (National Library of Medicine—neg. 58-381).

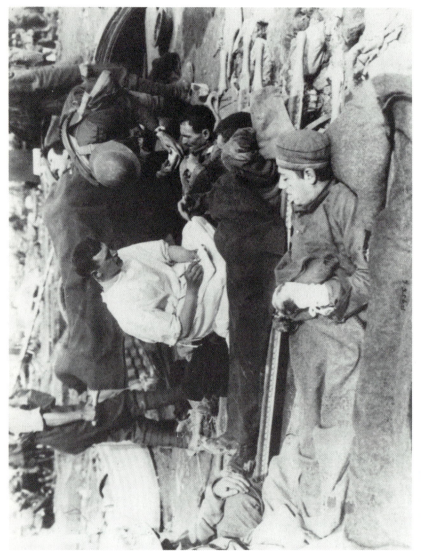

Fig. 3.124 The anti-war caption was written by Laurence Stallings, author of the famous play, *What Price Glory?* for Laurence Stallings, *The First War* (New York: Simon and Schuster, 1933) (Print owned by Stanley B. Burns, M.D., and the Burns Archive).

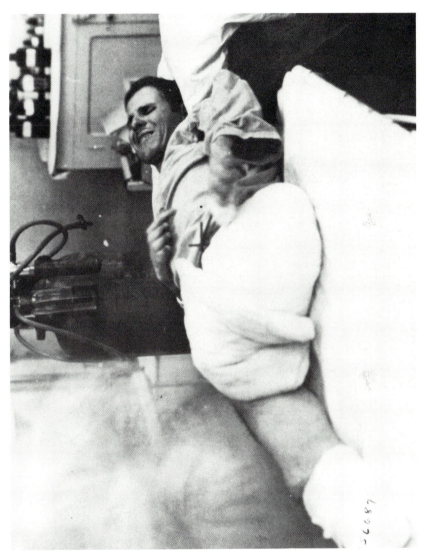

Fig. 3.125 World War I soldier: double amputee, c. 1918 (National Library of Medicine—United States Signal Corps).

CHAPTER IV

MULTIPLYING IMAGES, 1918-1939

In the interwar years, photography was one of the means by which the profession defined and advertised the role of medicine. Photographs showed contemporaries that medicine was vigorous, scientific, and a powerful agent of progress. This definition was gradually accepted by the public, which became familiar with the new imagery as it increasingly appeared in the press. The imagery in medical photographs corresponded to the medical profession's way of describing the world. Whether or not doctors were included in particular images, most people would have understood that doctors were the source of authority in medicine.

Medical photographs in these years were made in a variety of styles. The most modern styles, however, because they were employed by newspapers and magazines, were those that shaped the public perception of medicine. In these styles, an increasing number of photographs drew attention to particular people. By the mid-1930s, press photographers moved close to their subjects, and their attention to people was accompanied by a contraction of the space in which they viewed them.

During these years more medical pictures were taken in acute general hospitals than in any other setting. Wards, operating theaters, physical therapy departments and outpatient clinics were the most frequent photographic subjects. The visual model of hospital organization in British photographs ceased to be the great house. Wards were no longer depicted as domestic, but rather as they had been during the First World War and earlier in America—long, empty and symmetrical. Sometimes, pictures of wards looked like photographs of places of light industrial work (Fig. 4.1). Photographs of the same ward of a Liverpool hospital, taken in 1903 and 1930 (Figs. 4.2, 4.3), illustrate some aspects of this transformation. Domestic objects were no longer represented by the time the second photograph was taken. Patients were visible in the later photograph, although the nurses posed in much the same way as they did earlier. In most interwar pictures of wards, plants and flowers still appeared, although they were not usually as visibly luxuriant as they had been before the war. During the 1920s, when British voluntary hospitals experienced a financial crisis, photographs were often used for fund-raising purposes. Photographers at the Middlesex Hospital, for example, showed a modern looking ward, but with its ceiling supported by scaffolding (Fig. 4.4). The message was simple: modernity required cash. In these years, for the first time, British photographers also began to picture spartan, unadorned hospital wards in Poor Law hospitals (Fig. 4.5), which, however, resembled wards in voluntary institutions.

Photographs of American general hospitals continued to show clean, spacious, functional wards. Pictures taken in the 1920s and 1930s resemble those from the turn of the century (Figs. 4.6, 4.7). Wards for children were usually photographed as being as rigorously functional as those for adults. This photograph, however, represented the ward's mural decorations (Fig. 4.8).

Photographs of accommodation for private patients are rare in the archives of both countries. A British example depicted a ward in which patients were offered some domestic comfort and, more important, the opportunity for curtained privacy (Fig. 4.9). American hospitals in these years sometimes published photographs of empty rooms. These pictures, presumably, were composed to call attention to privacy in a medical institution and the comforts of contemporary domestic design (Fig. 4.10).

During the interwar years hospitals for people suffering from incurable diseases were still represented as domestic (Fig. 4.11). Sanatoria continued to be shown as inviting, sunny resorts (Fig. 4.12) and tuberculous patients remained subjects for portraits (Fig. 4.13). Sanatoria also advertised themselves as centers of medical and surgical intervention, notably by their employment of the artificial pneumothorax operation (Fig. 4.14).

By contrast with sanatoria, mental hospitals and their patients seem to have been photographed less frequently than before the war. Photographs representing asylums as great, self-contained, caring institutions almost ceased to be made in Britain. Pictures of psychiatric wards, even for children (Fig. 4.15), now resembled those taken in acute hospitals. This photograph, showing electrical therapy and massage being given to patients organized in groups, was unusual as a psychiatric representation, but very similar to the commonest images of general medicine (Fig. 4.16). Only a few non-clinical photographs of psychiatric patients seem to have been taken. A picture, taken in 1936, of a man being cared for in a padded cell was a close-up in the new style (Fig. 4.17).

American psychiatric patients in the interwar years were usually photographed seated in groups or performing menial tasks (Figs. 4.18, 4.19). Such work was regarded as important therapy for depressed patients. They were, however, rarely pictured as the recipients of medical treatment. The absence of a consistent image in photographs of institutional care for the mentally ill in both countries in these years is, presumably, explained by divisions within the psychiatric community.

Psychiatrists were losing confidence in custodial regimes and moral therapy, and the discipline was riven by disagreement among proponents of drug treatment, physical therapy, surgery, social psychiatry and psychoanalysis.

Nurses in hospitals were almost always photographed as people at work, as they had been during the war. By the mid-1930s the close-up was often employed for this purpose. This new style was, in part, related to the growing interest of contemporary photographers and their audiences in pictures of ordinary people at work. Lewis Hine in the United States and Emil Hoppé and later Bill Brandt in Britain were among the eminent photographers of the 1920s and 30s who made manual labor a photographic subject.[1] The disappearance of an image of nurses as passive was in part the result of this change in photography. It also followed from the new assertiveness of nurses as an occupational group, and of women in general. It was, in addition, part of the new image of medicine as interventive. The older image did not, however, disappear entirely (Fig. 4.20). Not surprisingly, new perceptions of the scientific role of hospitals and the redefinition of the nurse's job generated numerous photographs representing nursing students receiving education in science (Figs. 4.21, 4.22).

The work which nurses engaged in was increasingly depicted as very diverse. By the 1930s British nurses were photographed as doctors' assistants (Fig. 4.23), just as Americans had been two decades earlier. American nurses were sometimes represented treating patients without a doctor present (Fig. 4.24). They were also photographed performing tasks that remained invisible in Britain—giving an enema, for instance (Fig. 4.25), or participating in emergency care at a time when the medical emergency does not seem to have existed as a British photographic subject (Fig. 4.26). Some American nurses were depicted as managers (Fig. 4.27), and others were workers in pharmacies (Fig. 4.28) and laboratories (Fig. 4.29). In Britain, dispensing was often photographed as work performed by women, but it was not work for nurses (Fig. 4.30). On the other hand, British nurses, but apparently not their American counterparts, were depicted raising funds for hospitals. Such photographs sometimes used the image of the great institutional family (Fig. 4.31). By the 1930s, however, nurses began to be photographed raising funds for medical research, as well as for the hospital (Fig. 4.32).

The greater range of nurses' activities in American photographs may accord with a difference in actual work roles, but this cannot be simply deduced from the extant photographs. Other explanations are possible for these photographic differences. Nurses may have had greater power in American hospitals and thus had an increased likelihood of exerting some control over photographic representations. In addition, the American medical profession may have perceived nurses as more important than the British did.

The most frequent appearance of the working nurse was in photographs of technology. Before the war nurses were often depicted alongside machines. In the interwar years they were photographed using technology, particularly therapeutic apparatus (Fig. 4.33). Photographs like this proliferated in the interwar years. In the 1920s thousands of pictures were taken of large machines, particularly the apparatus used for electrical, radium and ultra-violet treatment (Figs. 4.34, 4.35).[2]

Photographs of nurses using such machines may have conjoined two images familiar to contemporaries. The first was the traditional one identifying the nurse with caring, which was now represented by work. The other was the visual image of science on the march, the language of which the public had learned from photographs and films of the day, particularly from pictures of rather glamorous and much publicized work in atomic and spectrum physics.[3] Thus medical photographs represented effective therapy, derived from science, given to individuals by caring people.

In Victorian pictures, women in uniform were nurses. In the 1930s, photographers working in the modern style began to represent nurses in uniform as women. One way in which this was done was to make them objects of sexual interest (Fig. 4.36). During the same years the nurse had already been accorded a sexual identity in films and popular literature.[4]

The image of the nurse in post-war years was created in association with a new image of the patient as a sick person. The patient's disease, the particular pathology, was usually represented away from public view with the techniques of clinical photography. Some photographs of disease, however, used other more familiar conventions. For instance, a boy in Kansas was photographed in 1921 before and after treatment with insulin (Fig. 4.37). Both pictures resembled the earliest clinical photographs in their use of extraneous clues to convey information about the boy's life. In the first, the boy's weakness was depicted by contrasting it with his mother's strength. After treatment, the boy's healthy physique— now dressed in a sailor shirt—filled the frame. His mother's absence might have suggested that the boy had achieved independence through medicine.

Patients were increasingly portrayed in the 1930s as individuals receiving care and attention. One notable British photograph from 1932 illustrates the conjuction of several themes we have been discussing. A *Daily Herald* photographer depicted cinema usherettes receiving sun-ray treatment, presumably to compensate for the hours they spent in darkness. At the left of the photograph, a nurse was in charge of both a lamp and the patients (Fig. 4.38). This image combined several elements: the use of new technology; the active, caring nurse; patients as people; humor; and the extension of medicine into ordinary life.

The new imagery represented medicine as legitimately extending beyond the immediate concerns of patients to their families and their working lives. In this American photograph, mothers and children waited in a hospital social service office (Fig. 4.39). In this British one a white-coated almoner interviewed a patient (Fig. 4.40).

During the interwar years photographs of familiar subjects were composed in new ways. This was partly because the pictures were used to convey alternative and additional meanings. Although the poor were still required to wait, they were no longer faceless. In waiting room photographs of the 1930s, hospital personnel were not in attendance as they were in pre-war pictures. Photographers drew attention to individuals in the crowd, and contrived humorous pictures of waiting patients: for example, note the sign at the top of this picture in which the most prominent individual was a boy (Fig. 4.41).

A comparison of two photographs of waiting patients exemplifies how a great photographer composed a picture to make a statement about medicine. An anonymous British photographer depicted patients waiting on hospital stairs and crowding through the door of a clinic. The picture was taken from the consultant's viewpoint at the top of the stairs (Fig. 4.42). Edward Steichen, the American photographer, in a photograph he titled "On the Clinic Stairs" showed patients looking upward toward a light (Fig. 4.43). Both of these pictures identified waiting as a common experience, but Steichen was probably signalling that medicine was the light to which people in darkness should look.[5]

Most medical photographs were taken in places that were dependent on philanthropic and public funds. In this typical British picture the patient acknowledged the patronage of the church and royalty (Fig. 4.44). The nurse was represented in a posture conventional in the presence of august personages. Photographs of British patients with their benefactors were widely published. In Chapter I we described two curious representations of American philanthropists in a children's ward (Figs. 4.45, 4.46). In one they stood in a group, in the other the woman read a book to a young patient. Philanthropy at the bedside was not a frequent photographic subject in America.

In Britain, a visit by royalty to a hospital was always an occasion to be photographed. Such pictures were used to confirm and celebrate the role of the hospital in national life. Even the crown, however, could be represented as taking second place to scientific patient care (Fig. 4.47). For example, in this picture taken in 1939 at the opening of the new Westminster hospital, the King and the Queen were photographed, uncharacteristically, with their backs turned, inspecting an X-ray as it was described by a doctor.

The doctor with the King and Queen in this photograph is one of the few to have appeared in this chapter. Although doctors had become the most powerful figures in the medical world, they did not cultivate photographic visibility.[6] Except for the rituals of surgery, there were very few photographs of doctors treating patients. Private patients were never photographed, as far as we know. Most of the few photographs of doctors with patients that we have seen were taken in outpatient clinics or, less often, on ward rounds. The relative absence of pictures of consultations suggests that a public imagery was not compatible with the profession's strong commitment to the confidentiality of the private medical encounter.

The hospital doctors who were photographed with public patients were almost invariably engaged in some activity. The majority of these photographs represented diagnosis as the crucial moment for doctors and patients. Children continued to have low photographic status, as in this picture of a surgical outpatient clinic in which the surgeon had the familiar sterilizer in front of him (Fig. 4.48). A photograph of a British medical outpatient clinic in 1924 depicted four physicians (or students) in coats and ties observing while a white-coated colleague examined a half-naked man. This was a representation of a public examination of a member of one class by members of another. No contemporary viewer could possibly have confused the picture with one of a private consultation in Harley Street, if any existed (Fig. 4.49).

In 1939, *Picture Post* published a photograph of a private medical encounter in order to depict the apotheosis of the English doctor (Fig. 4.50). In it, Thomas, later Lord, Horder, the King's physician, sat in what the magazine described as the "most famous consulting room in the world."[7] The "patient" was undoubtedly an actor playing the part. Although Horder was an exceptionally able clinical scientist, in this his most public moment he was photographed as a man of cultured gentility without a single visual reminder of his professional expertise.

Unlike British hospital doctors, when American doctors and their patients were photographed, they did not appear to be in public arenas. Other patients and medical workers—except occasionally nurses—were rarely included in these photographs, as they rountinely would have been before the war. The pictures were composed to portray personal relationships (Fig. 4.51).[8] During these years, not surprisingly, the American Medical Association was insisting vigorously that everyone should have a personal doctor.

In America, where medical education and training were more highly organized than in Britain, photographs of it were frequently taken, especially in amphiteaters (Fig. 4.52). The few comparable British photographs usually depicted small groups of students in clinics (Fig. 4.53).

Imagery that contemporaries would have associated with science increasingly appeared in American and British portrayals of hospital medicine. Photographs of hospital medicine had a scientific appearance, but displayed no imagery of a specific *medical* science. Few publically available pictures were taken of the practice of medical research and basic science. Such pictures were usually placed in private albums or in the archives of learned societies. This picture of the physiologist Walter B. Cannon, at work in his laboratory, was given as a souvenir to his postgraduate students at the Harvard Medical School (Fig. 4.54). Presumably, such pictures were used to celebrate the basic sciences among practitioners, rather than to popularize the disciplines. Antivivisectionist sentiment no doubt contributed to this reticence. More important, we suspect that because the medical profession identified the hospital as the visual embodiment of progress, so did the public. Before the 1950s, only a few photographs represent laboratory research as the source of medical progress. *Life*, for example, depicted the first American clinical research center for chronic disease in photographs of patients receiving treatment using new technology.[9] Research laboratories were, however, sometimes photographed in political contexts (Fig. 4.55).

In America between the wars, the scientific character of medical progress was most frequently represented by the photography of surgery. Over a generation conventions had been created for photographing surgery. By the 1920s, surgeons and their assistants were frequently viewed through a camera placed above the operating table or sometimes at the top of an amphitheater filled with spectators. During the same years in which the personalities of patients in the wards began to be represented in photographs, surgical patients became almost indistinguishable from the equipment and sterile sheets which surrounded them.

In 1929 Steichen, employing his characteristic style, transformed the surgical photograph into a picture of an awesome, dramatic event. Using the familiar conventions of surgical photography, Steichen created a powerful image which he called "Death Takes a Holiday." The title was that of a contemporary play which was later made into a successful film (Fig. 4.56). The photograph was taken from the angle of someone high in the amphitheater. The patient's body was implied by the positions of the surgeons and the anesthetist. Distractions, such as the buckets in the left foreground, were immersed in deep shadow, unlike those in the operation of 1888 at the Massachusetts General Hospital described in Chapter III, (Fig. 3.79). Like the play from which Steichen took his caption, surgery was a performance which an audience observed from a distance.

Steichen's photograph helped to transform the surgical image into a cliché in both formal medical pictures and in popular culture. His image was frequently imitated by professional photographers working in hospitals (Fig. 4.57). It was also used in the theatre and in films. In 1933, Lee Strassberg, the eminent theatrical director, used Steichen's vision as a stage set for his prize-winning production of Sidney Kingsley's *Men in White*, a play about the heroism of doctors and the power of modern medicine (Fig. 4.58).[10]

Although photographs of surgery were routinely included in albums and other commemorations of British hospitals in these years, fewer pictures of it were taken than in the United States. Therapeutic technology—especially the Finsen Lamp, the iron lung, and large electrical apparatus—appeared more often in medical photographs. Most of the British photographs of surgery used the conventions we have described, representing surgery as a theater with performers and spectators. However, in a number of photographs of British surgery the communication of drama was of negligible importance (Fig. 4.59).

The dominance of hospital medicine effectively deprived public health practitioners of power. Surgeons had created a public imagery that exalted their place in the medical world. Earlier in the century, public health practitioners had also begun to create a distinct imagery of themselves and their work. They barely modified this imagery in the 1920s and 1930s. Medicine had changed but representations of public health had not. In most photographs of public health work in schools and clinics people, usually children, were examined, vaccinated, weighed, taught, or supervised in group activity. A picture of a school clinic in London in 1938 (Fig. 4.60) had much in common with earlier photographs (Fig. 3.111, for example).

Many photographs of public health work in these years represented medicine as responsible for individual and familial physical and psychological well-being. A persistent theme in most of these pictures was the rearing of healthy children. Families, and particularly mothers, were photographed receiving supervision and guidance from doctors and nurses (Fig. 4.61, 4.62). By the late 1930s the new style was employed to create what eventually became a familiar image (Fig. 4.63). The close-up made the child's well-being an integral part of a familial relationship. Similarly, advocacy of contraception was confirmed by using medical imagery (Figs. 4.64, 4.65).

Photographs of men in public health settings often depicted venereal disease being detected or treated. In an American photograph, a test for syphilis was conducted on a sidewalk by a doctor and a nurse (Fig. 4.66). Such photographs were yet another representation of medical concern for the health of children and families.

The new medical imagery we have described in this chapter became commonplace in the years between the wars. Photographs of hospitals, of technology, of nurses and patients—and of all of them together—appeared with increasing frequency in newspapers and magazines. These pictures were normative. They created expectations of what medical care should be and they showed people how to behave in medical encounters. Photography was one of the means by which medicine made itself distinctive—a specialized technical occupation, but simultaneously a caring activity.

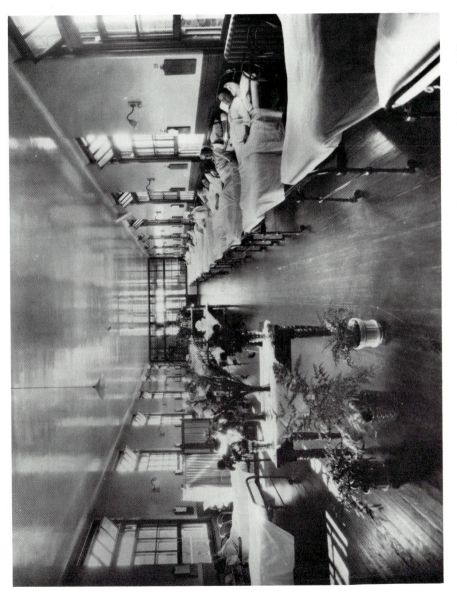

Fig. 4.1 St. James's Hospital, Balham, London, 1930. The absence of nurses at work is unusual (Greater London Photograph Library—81/9368).

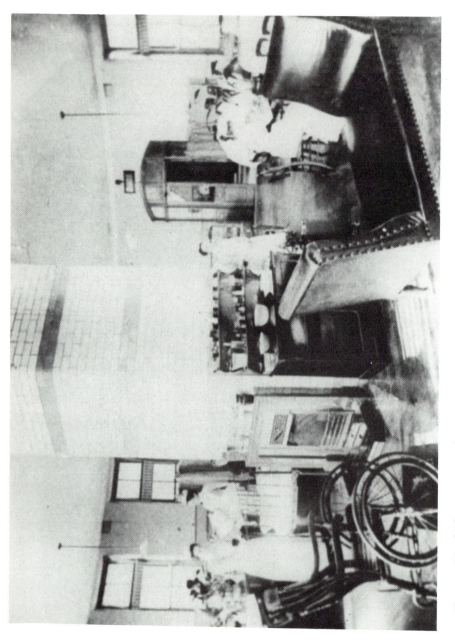

Fig. 4.2 Ward Three, Liverpool's Northern Hospital, 1902 (Courtesy of Dr. T. Cook).

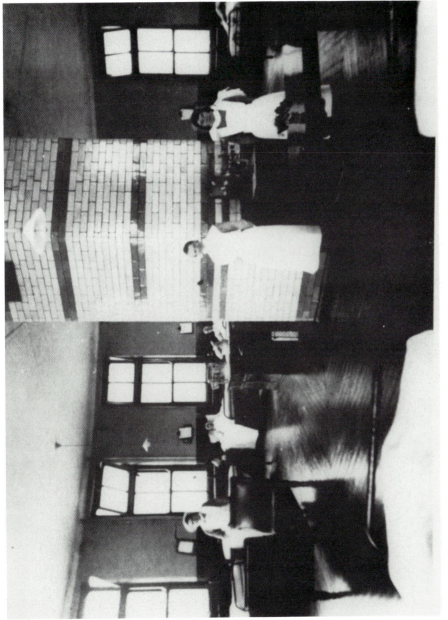

Fig. 4.3 The same, 1930, the nurses are posed as in the earlier picture (Courtesy of Dr. T. Cook).

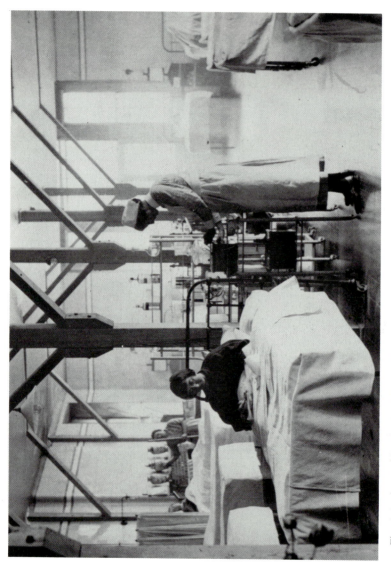

Fig. 4.4 A ward in the Middlesex Hospital, London, c. 1925. The hospital produced a large number of photographs during its fund raising campaign. This is a representation of modern medicine operating in times of financial stringency. Note the nurse at work, at what appears to be a surgical dressing trolley. Compare with Fig. 3.85 (The Archivist of The Middlesex Hospital).

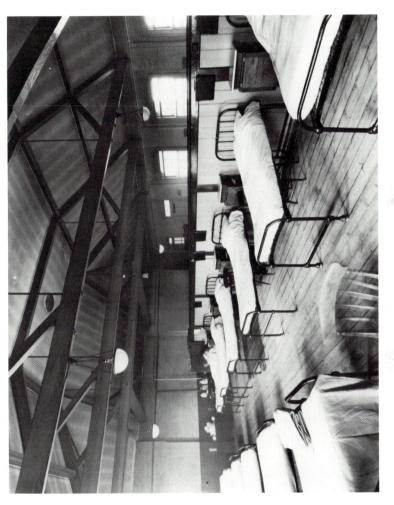

Fig. 4.5 Lambeth Hospital, 1933. Like St. James's Balham (Fig. 4.1) this was an old Poor Law Hospital, which became a Municipal Hospital run by the London County Council. The use of this photograph remains conjectural. Was it produced to advertise simple but adequate care, or condemn the provision of bare necessities? (Greater London Photograph Library—84/430).

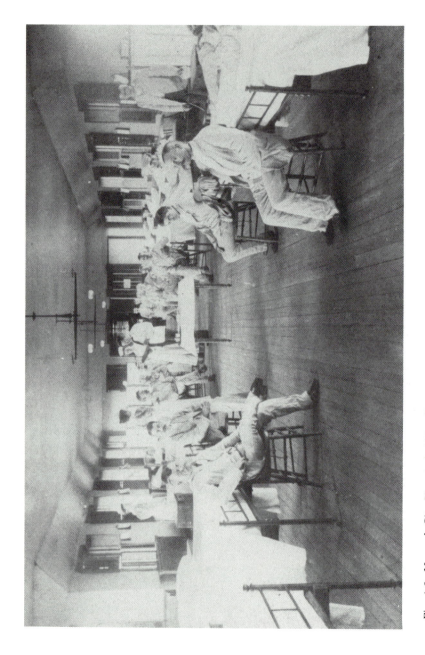

Fig. 4.6 Newark City Hospital, 1895. Compare this photograph with Fig. 4.7 (University of Medicine and Dentistry of New Jersey, George F. Smith Library—PC-24/78).

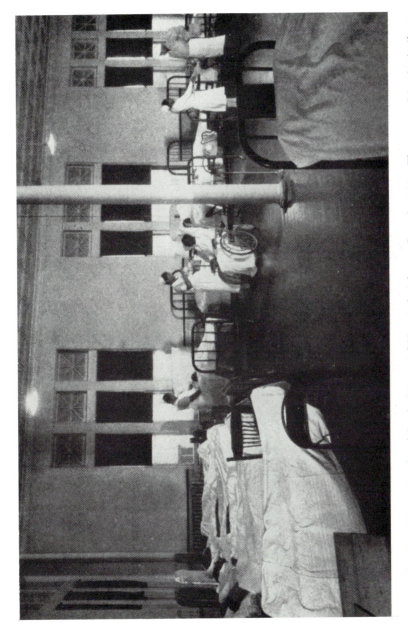

Fig. 4.7 The "Negro Ward" of Grady Memorial Hospital, Atlanta, Georgia, 1934. The composition is similar to photographs of nineteenth-century wards (Grady Memorial Hospital, Atlanta, Georgia).

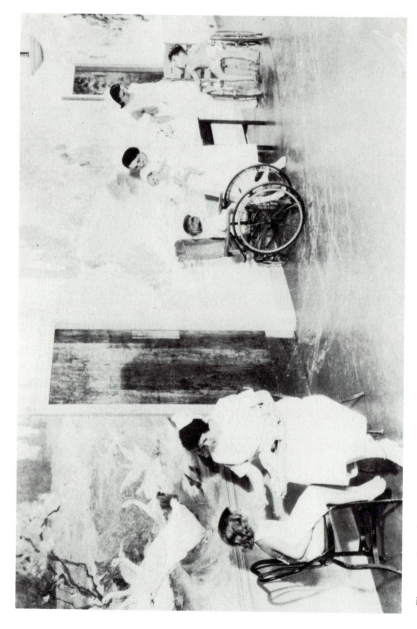

Fig. 4.8 A pediatric ward at Grady Memorial Hospital in Atlanta, Georgia, 1936 (Grady Memorial Hospital, Atlanta, Georgia).

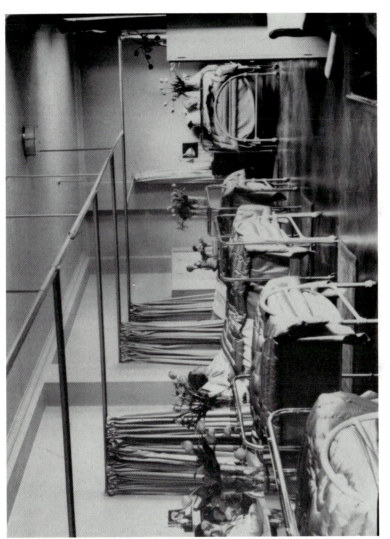

Fig. 4.9 Woolavington Wing, the Middlesex Hospital, 1935. This was a private wing built after a bequest by Lord Woolavington and opened in 1934. The wing provided for middle class patients, too well off to be admitted among the poor, yet with insufficient means to pay for treatment in a private nursing home. The picture represents just that—a degree of comfort in a relatively public space (The Archivist of The Middlesex Hospital).

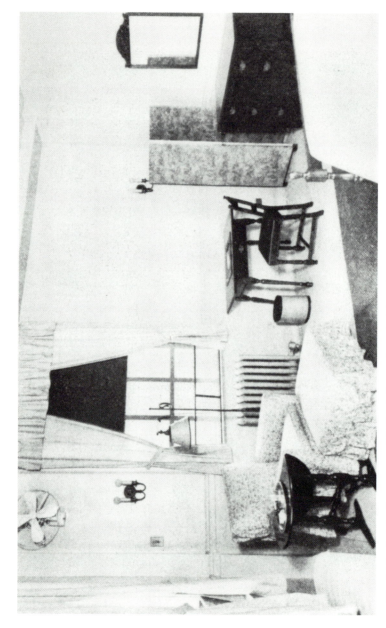

Fig. 4.10 A private room at Michael Reese Hospital in Chicago in the 1930s (Michael Reese Hospital and Medical Center, Chicago, Illinois).

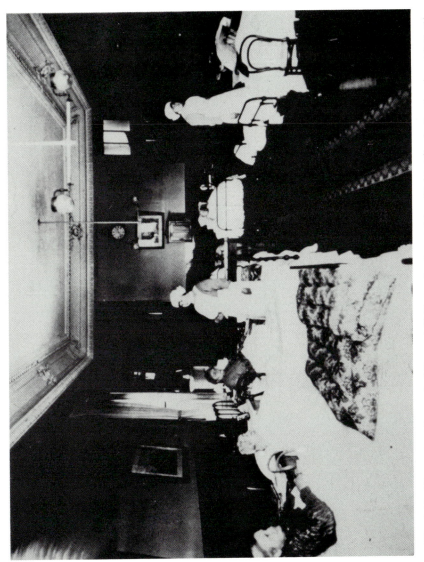

Fig. 4.11 The women's ward of Broomhill Home for Incurables, Kirkintilloch, Scotland, c. 1925. The significance of domesticity, of course, is that people die at home, as it were, not in hospital (Greater Glasgow Health Board Archives).

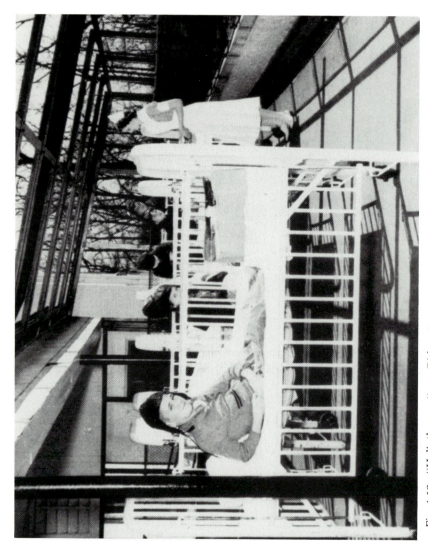

Fig. 4.12 "Heliotherapy" at Ridge Farm, a tuberculosis sanatorium affiliated with St. Louis Children's Hospital in the 1920s (Washington University, School of Medicine Library—80-9861).

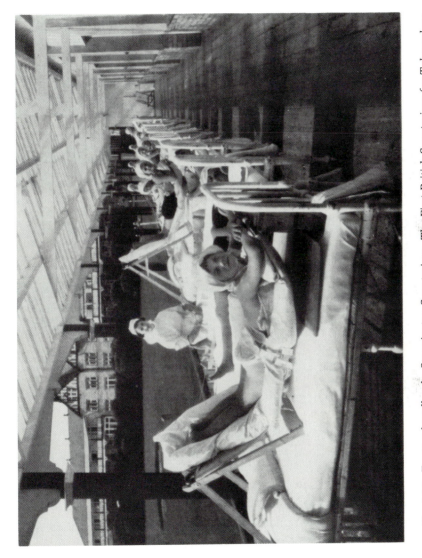

Fig. 4.13 From a handbook, *Stannington Sanatorium. The First British Sanatorium for Tuberculous Children,* n.d. [1936?] The guidebook advertised the outdoor life of the sanatorium and the scientific diagnosis and therapy available (Wellcome Institute Library, London).

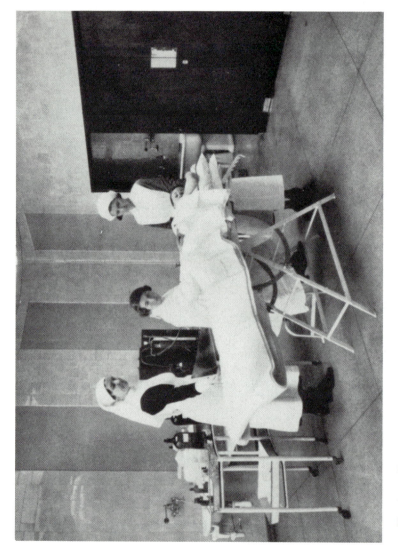

Fig. 4.14 From the same handbook as Fig. 4.13 (Wellcome Institute Library, London).

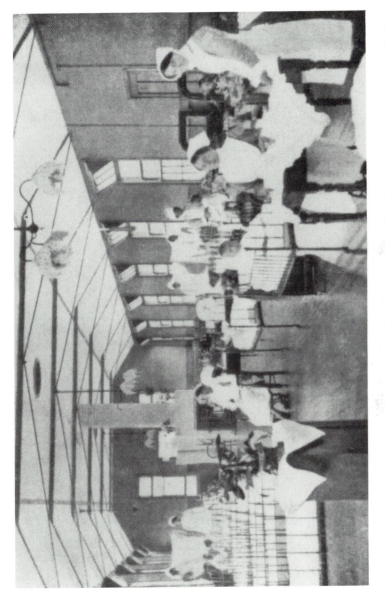

Fig. 4.15 A photograph entitled 'A Typical Children's Ward at a Mental Hospital' from Sir A. Powell, *The Metropolitan Asylums Board and its Work 1867-1930* (London: The Board, 1930) facing p. 46. The change from the concept of the institutions as a home for the insane to a hospital was embodied in the 1930 *Mental Treatment Act*, when asylum was dropped from official use in favor of mental hospital (Wellcome Institute Library, London).

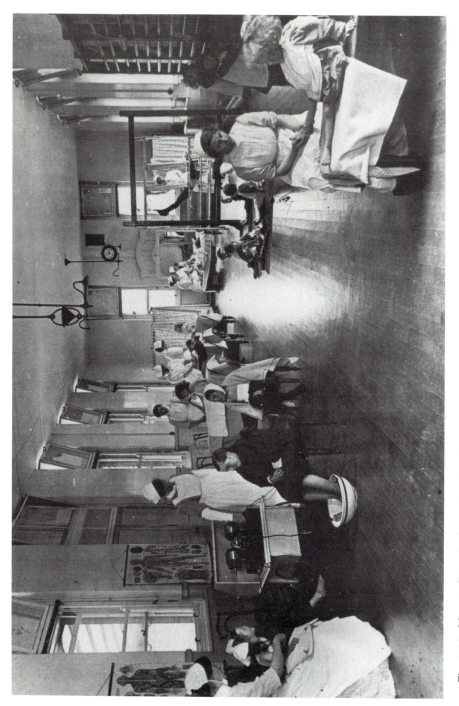

Fig. 4.16 Metropolitan Asylums Board, c. 1930 (Sport and General Press Agency).

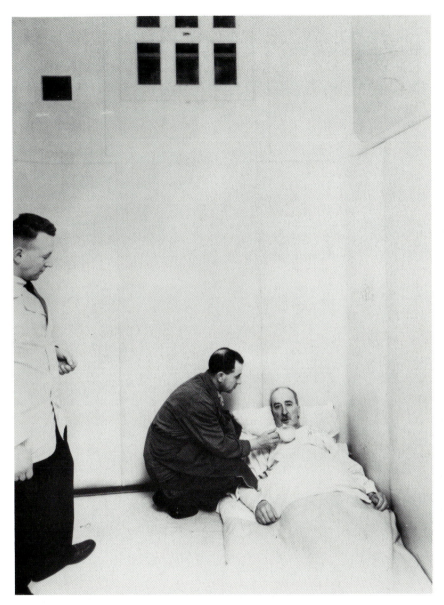

Fig. 4.17 A padded cell, Constance Road Institution, London, 1936. This is a typical thirties rather than twenties picture, it is a close-up approach. Again we have no indication that this picture was not used to stigmatize the violently mad. But its conventional construction suggests its purpose was to represent personal care (Greater London Photograph Library—80/7381).

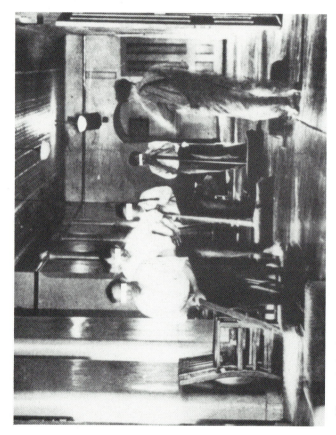

Fig. 4.18 Patients polishing a hallway floor, Elgin State Hospital, 1930s (John C. Burnham and Elgin Mental Health Center).

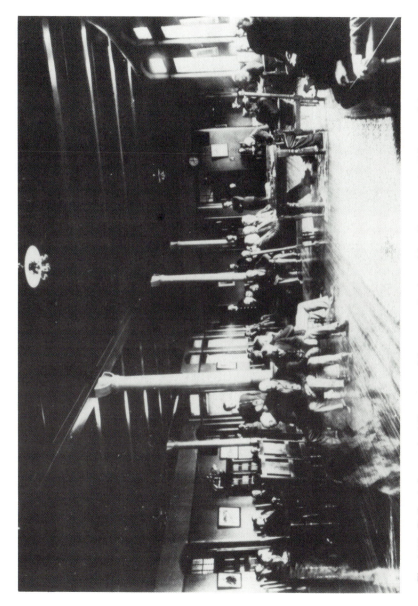

Fig. 4.19 Patients in men's sitting room, Mateawan Asylum, New Jersey, 1920 (Library of Congress—Bain Collection).

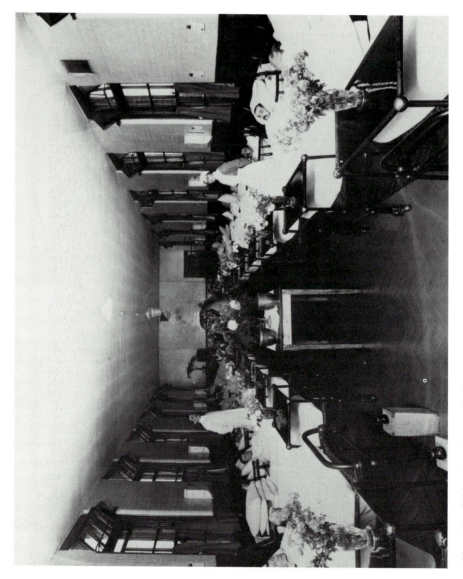

Fig. 4.20 Male chronic ward, Hammersmith Hospital, 1936 (Greater London Photograph Library—84/434)

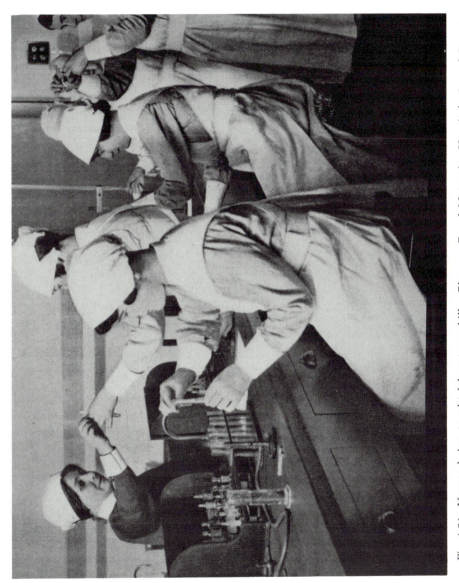

Fig. 4.21 Nurses being taught laboratory skills. Glasgow Royal Maternity Hospital, *Annual Report*, 1927 (Greater Glasgow Health Board Archives).

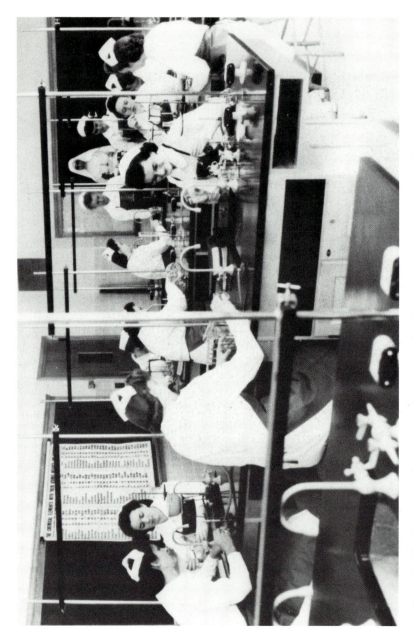

Fig. 4.22 Student nurses in a science laboratory, St. Mary's School of Nursing, Madison, Wisconsin, 1930. A nun presides over the laboratory at rear right of the photograph (St. Mary's Hospital Medical Center, Madison, Wisconsin).

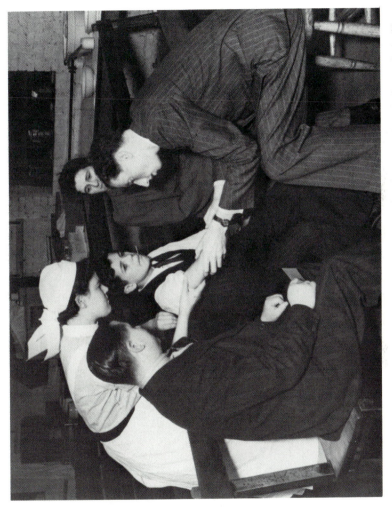

Fig. 4.23 Casualty (Emergency) Department, St. Bartholomew's hospital, c. 1940. The intimacy of the shot is once again characteristic of the late 1930s, as is the representation of medicine as caring for families. (Compare this with the stringent visiting hours for inpatients and the ban on visitors under fourteen years of age at about the same time. See Fig. 5.7) (Department of Medical Illustration, St. Bartholomew's Hospital).

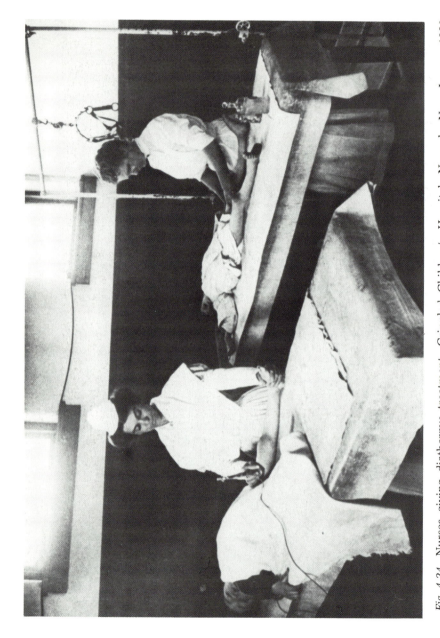

Fig. 4.24 Nurses giving diathermy treatment, Crippled Children's Hospital, Newark, New Jersey, 1920 (Newark Public Library).

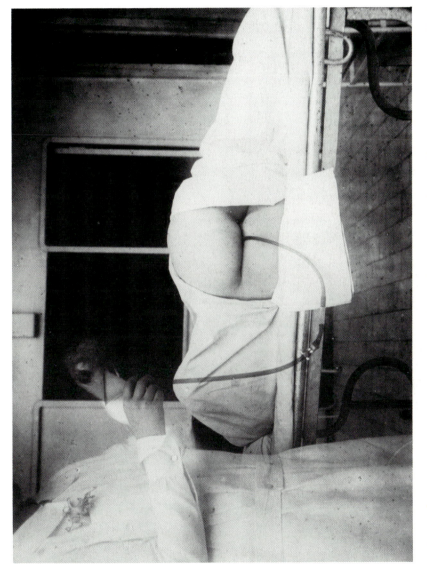

Fig. 4.25 Administering an enema at New York Hospital in the 1920s (Medical Archives, New York Hospital—Cornell Medical Center).

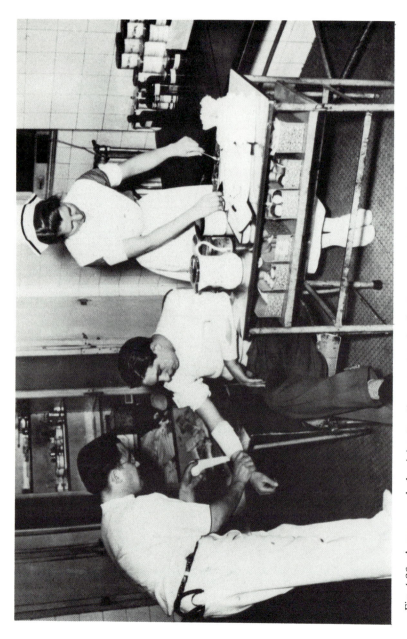

Fig. 4.26 A nurse and physician treating a patient in the Emergency Room of Newark City Hospital, Newark, New Jersey, in the mid-1930s (University Medicine and Dentistry of New Jersey, George F. Smith Library—PC-22/3). Compare with the similar composition of Fig. 4.23, which is not a picture about an emergency.

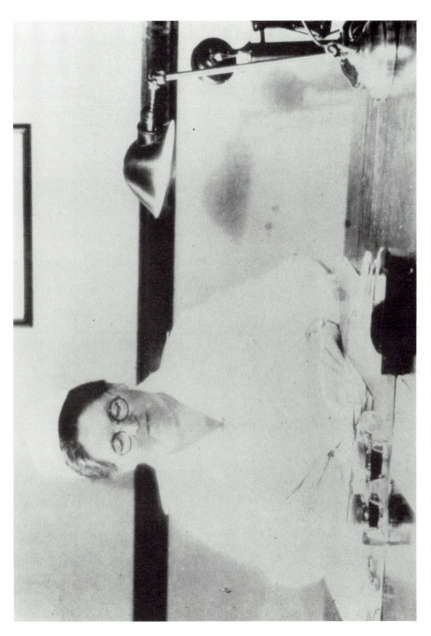

Fig. 4.27 Director of nursing, Gillette State Hospital for Crippled Children, St. Paul, Minnesota, 1935 (Gillette Children's Hospital, St. Paul, Minnesota).

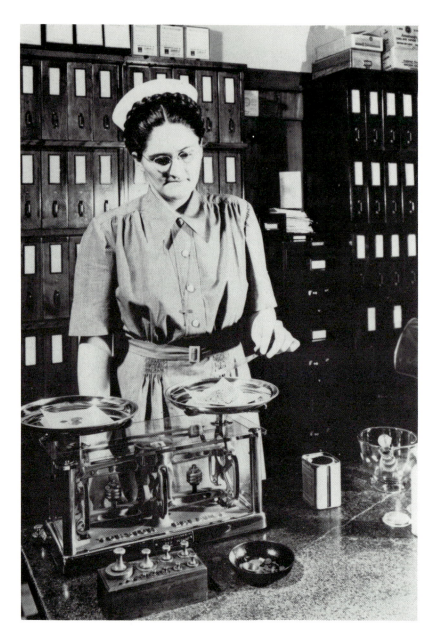

Fig. 4.28 Sister Gladys Robinson, the first director of the hospital pharmacy at Milwaukee Hospital, Wisconsin, c. 1925 (Good Samaritan Medical Center, Milwaukee, Wisconsin).

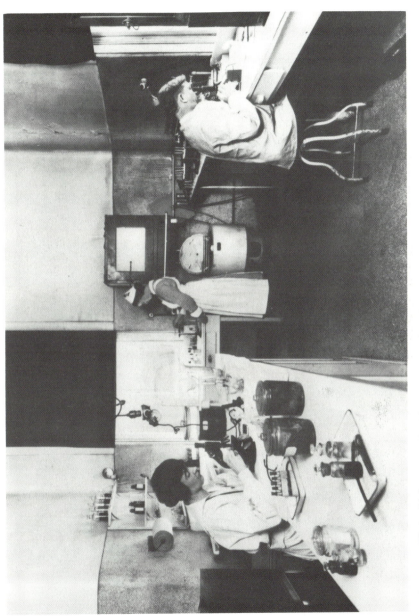

Fig. 4.29 Clinical laboratory, St. Vincent Hospital, Indianapolis, Indiana, 1923 (St. Vincent Hospital and Health Care Center, Indianapolis, Indiana).

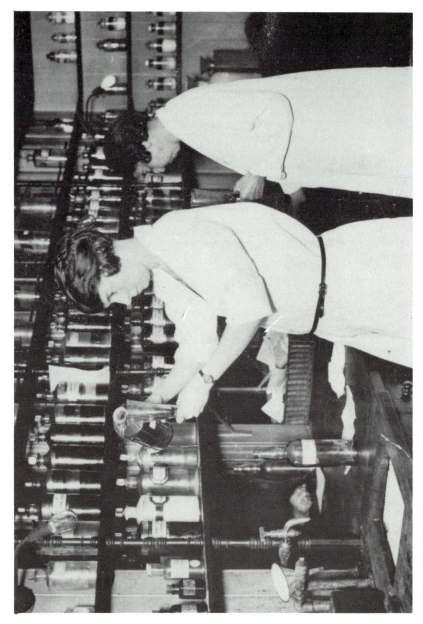

Fig. 4.30 The dispensary, the Middlesex Hospital, n.d., c. 1925 (The Archivist of the Middlesex Hospital).

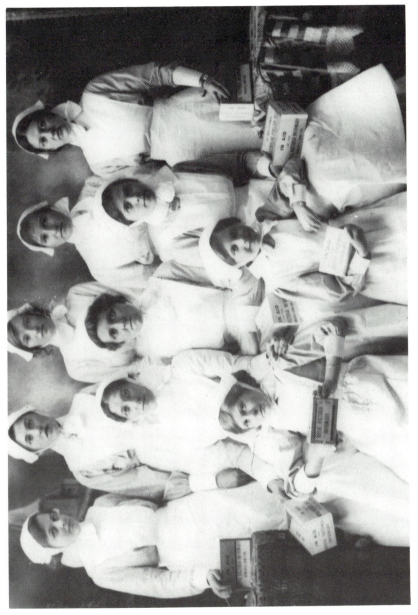

Fig. 4.31 Nurses collecting for the Royal Victoria Infirmary at Newcastle, n.d. (Beamish North of England Open Air Museum, Durham n16795).

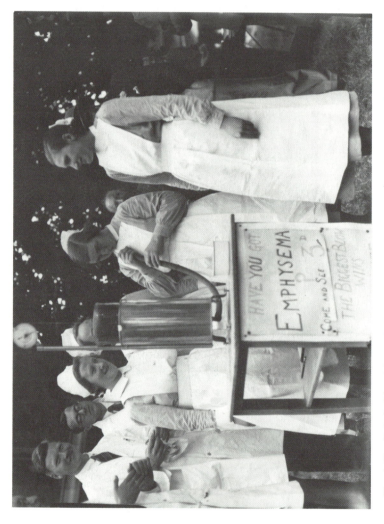

Fig. 4.32 Gala held at King's College Hospital, Denmark Hill, June 1937. Note the familiar connection between science and large clinical machinery. Compare also the similar, and almost contemporary, depiction of nurses and doctors in Fig. 5.8 (Syndication International [1986] Ltd.)

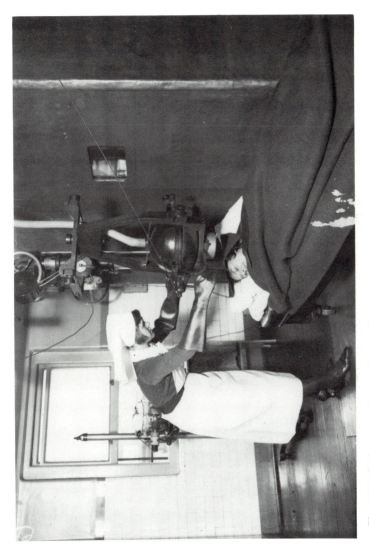

Fig. 4.33 Patient receiving X-ray therapy at Charing Cross Hospital 1932 (Syndication International [1986] Ltd.).

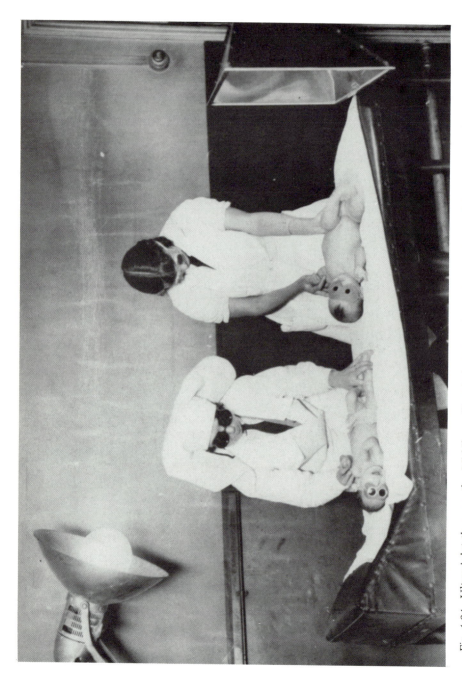

Fig. 4.34 Ultraviolet therapy, the Middlesex Hospital, 1931 (The Archivist of the Middlesex Hospital).

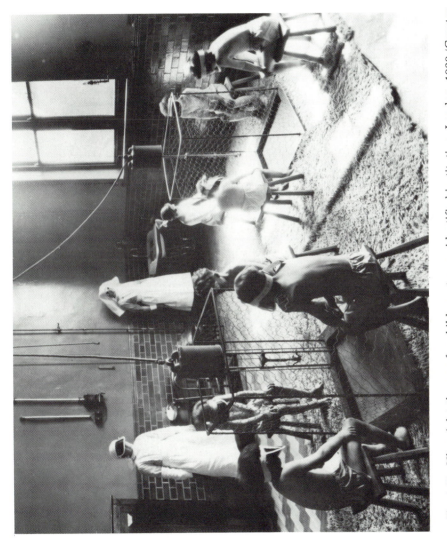

Fig. 4.35 Ultraviolet therapy for children at an unidentified institution, London, 1930 (Greater London Photograph Library—84/416).

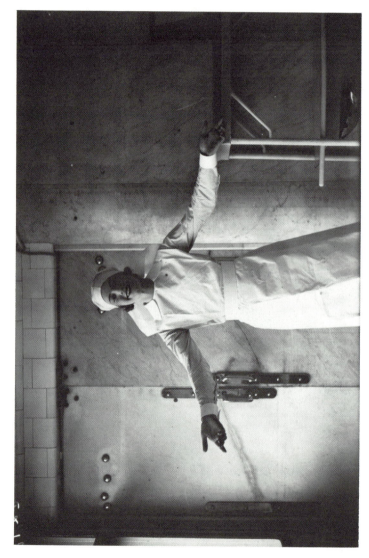

Fig. 4.36 Nurse appealing for funds for Charing Cross Hospital, c. 1933 (Syndication International [1986] Ltd.).

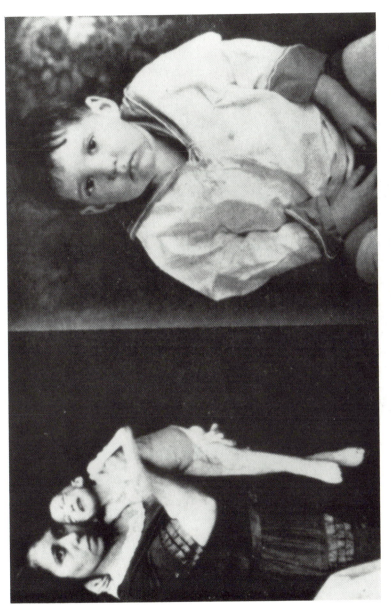

Fig. 4.37 The treatment of diabetes at the University of Kansas Hospital, Kansas City, c. 1925 (University of Kansas Medical Center, Department of the History and Philosophy of Medicine. Reproduced with permission from the *Journal of the Kansas Medical Society*).

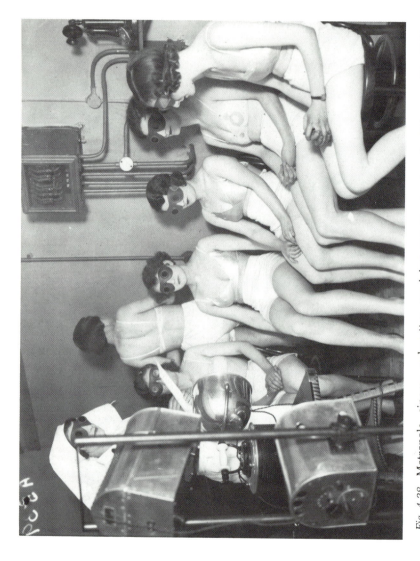

Fig. 4.38 Metropole cinema usherettes receiving sun-ray treatment, February 20, 1932 (Syndication International [1986] Ltd.).

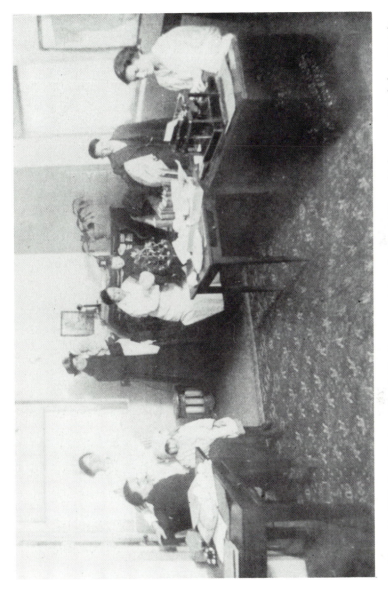

Fig. 4.39 This is a photograph, similar to many taken in the 1920s, which represented the space in which medical work took place. Compare the depiction of personal care, typical of the 1920s, in Fig. 4.40 (United Hospital Fund, 1917).

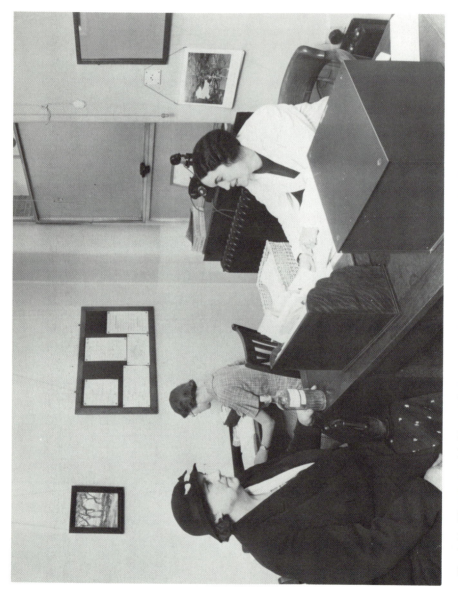

Fig. 4.40 Hammersmith Hospital almoner's office, 1936 (Greater London Photograph Library—81/9365).

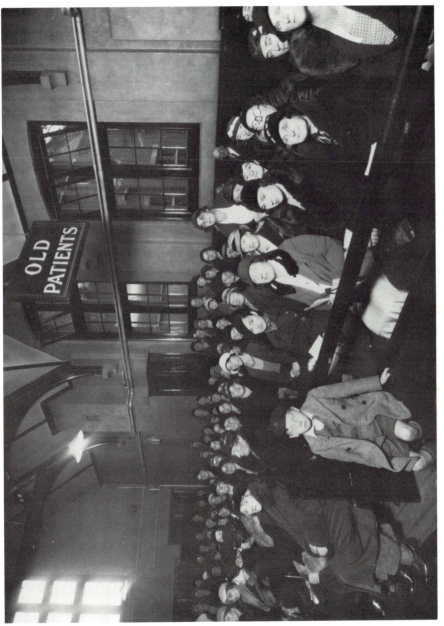

Fig. 4.41 The German Hospital, London, n.d., interwar years (Department of Medical Illustration, St. Bartholomew's Hospital).

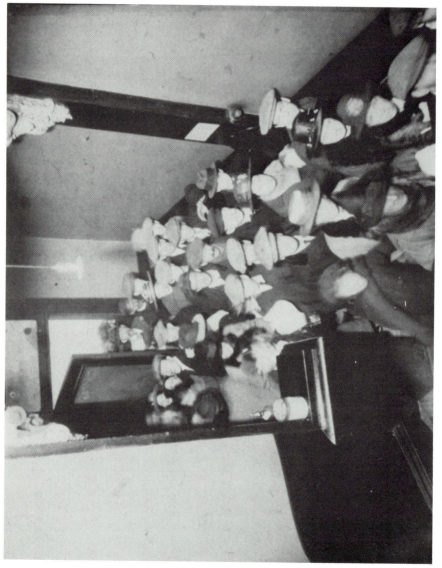

Fig. 4.42 Out-patients, Glasgow, Ear Nose and Throat Hospital, 1930 (Greater Glasgow Health Board Archives).

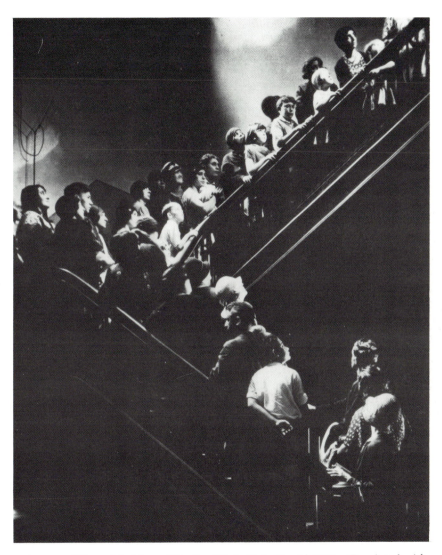

Fig. 4.43 Edward Steichen, ''On the Clinic Stairs'' mid-1920s (Reprinted with the permission of Joanna L. Steichen).

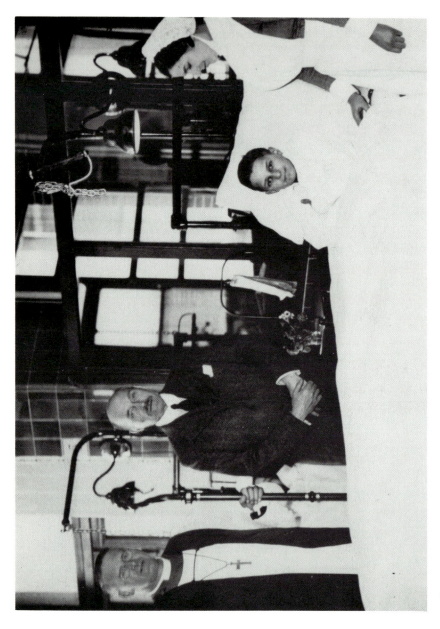

Fig. 4.44 Prince Arthur of Connaught opens the Bond St. Ward, the Middlesex Hospital, April 23, 1936 (The Archivist of The Middlesex Hospital).

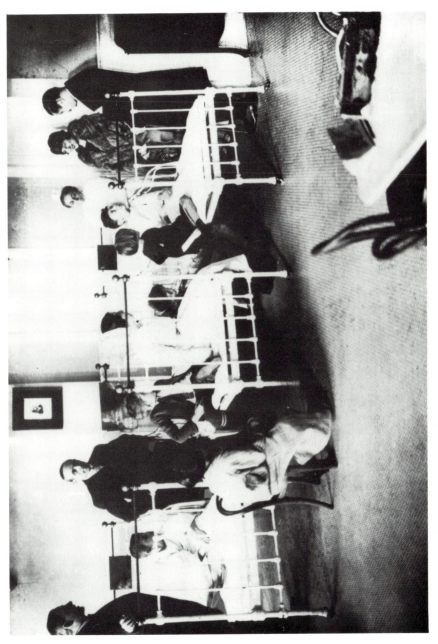

Fig. 4.45 Children's ward, New York Post-Graduate Hospital, 1920 (Library of Congress—Bain Collection).

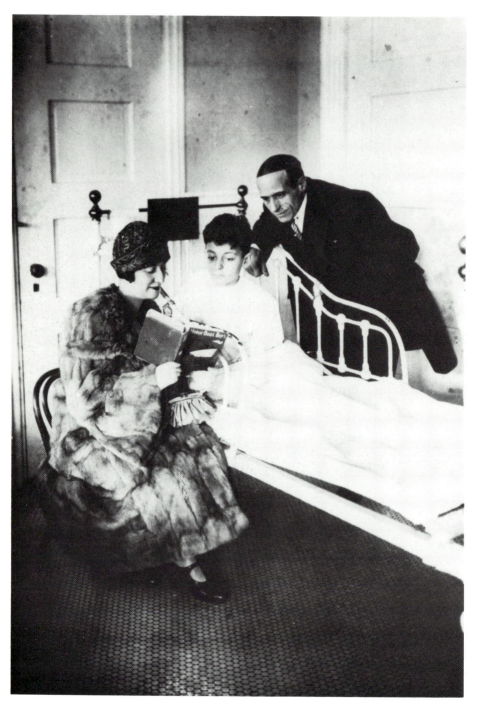

Fig. 4.46 Reading to the child at the far right in Fig. 4.45 (Library of Congress—Bain Collection).

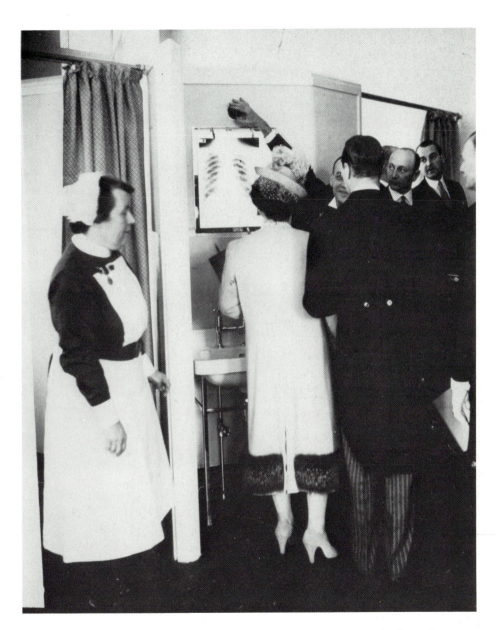

Fig. 4.47 Press photograph of King George VI and Queen Elizabeth at the Westminster Hospital after an opening ceremony, April 20, 1939 (Riverside Health Authority).

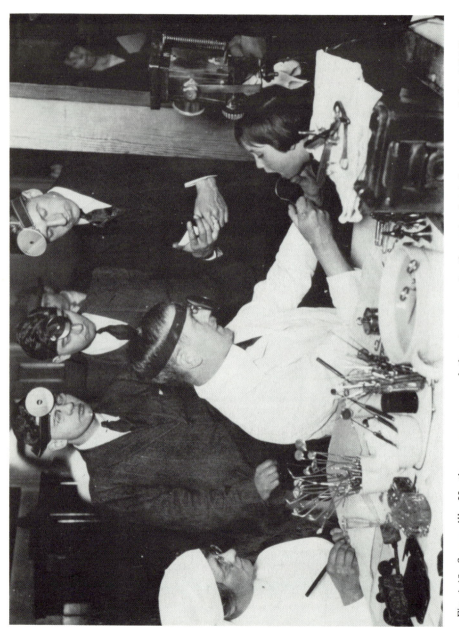

Fig. 4.48 Somerville Hastings, ear, nose and throat surgeon in the outpatient department of the Middlesex Hospital, c. 1924 (The Archivist of The Middlesex Hospital).

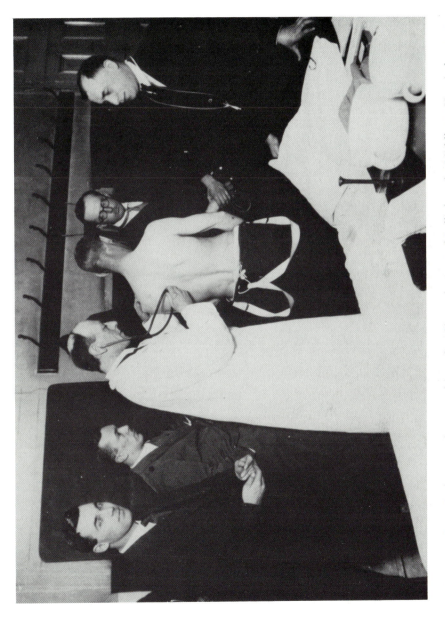

Fig. 4.49 E. A. Cockayne, who was educated at Charterhouse and Balliol, at the Middlesex Hospital, c. 1924. Cockayne was related to the aristocracy through his mother's second marriage (The Archivist of The Middlesex Hospital).

237

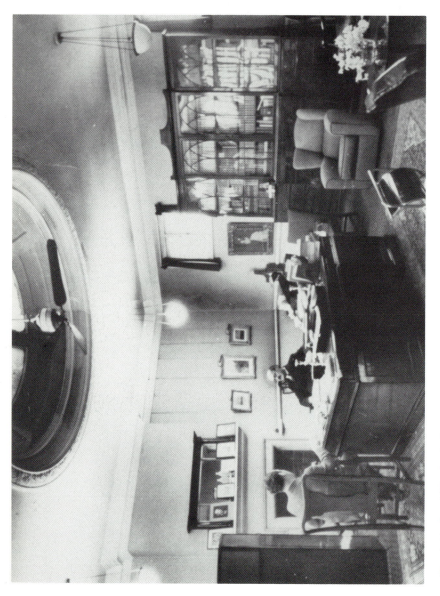

Fig. 4.50 Lord Horder in his Harley Street rooms in a center page spread in *Picture Post* which described Horder as having 'a big brain, penetrating eyes and a shrewd power of diagnosis.' *Picture Post*, December 2, 1939, pp. 26-27 (BBC, Hulton Picture Library).

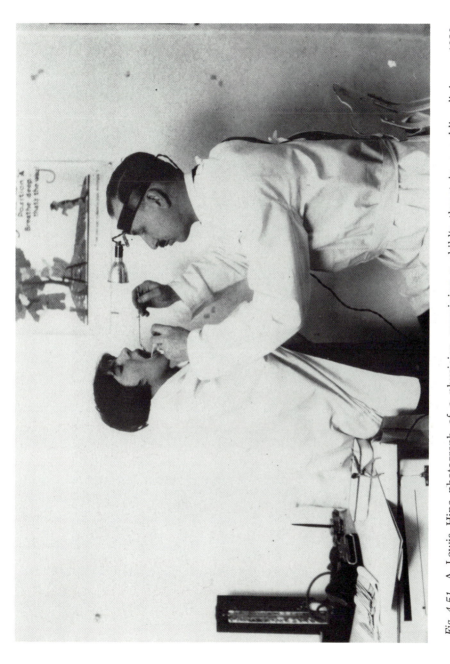

Fig. 4.51 A Lewis Hine photograph of a physician examining a child's throat in a public clinic, c. 1920 (International Museum of Photography, Eastman House, Rochester, New York).

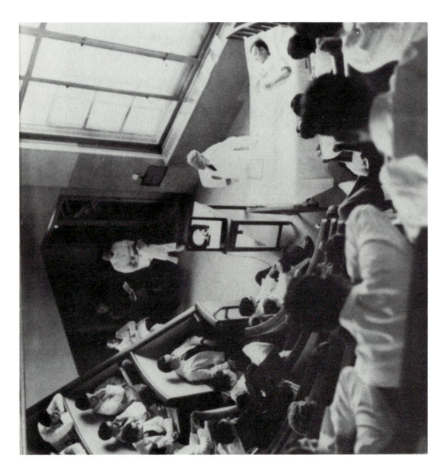

Fig. 4.52 Surgical grand rounds at New York Hospital, 1936. Representations of this sort seem to have been rare in Britain (Medical Archives, New York Hospital—Cornell Medical Center—neg. 25).

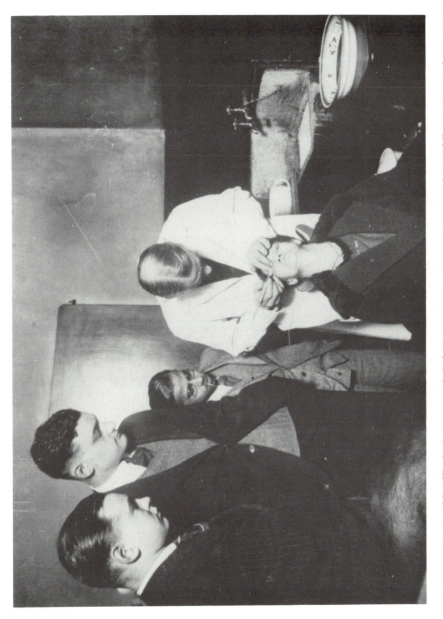

Fig. 4.53 Reginald Affleck Greeves, ophthalmic surgeon, in out-patients at the Middlesex Hospital, c. 1925. Judging by the rather shabby background, this picture was probably taken as part of the fund raising campaign (The Archivist of The Middlesex Hospital).

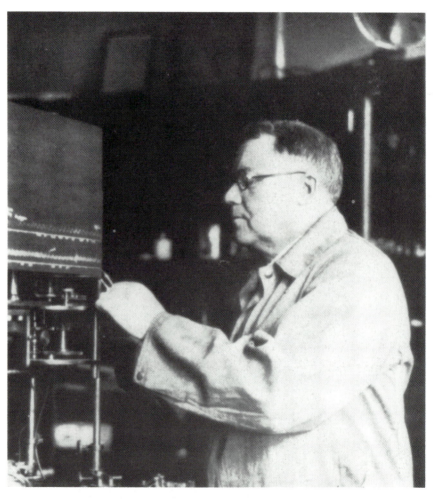

Fig. 4.54 Walter B. Cannon in his laboratory at the Harvard Medical School in the mid-1930s (Collection of Dr. John Romano, University of Rochester School of Medicine and Dentistry).

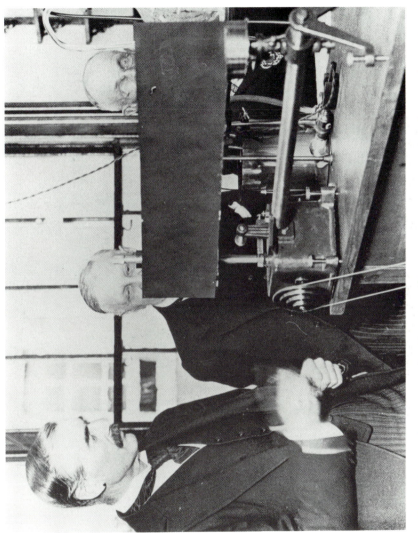

Fig. 4.55 Neville Chamberlain, Minister of Health, at the opening of the Pharmacology Laboratories of the University of London's School of Pharmacy, June 16, 1926. This picture sanctioned medical research and testified that there were progressive, scientifically aware elements in the Conservative party (*The Pharmaceutical Journal and Pharmacist, 1926, 116:645.*)

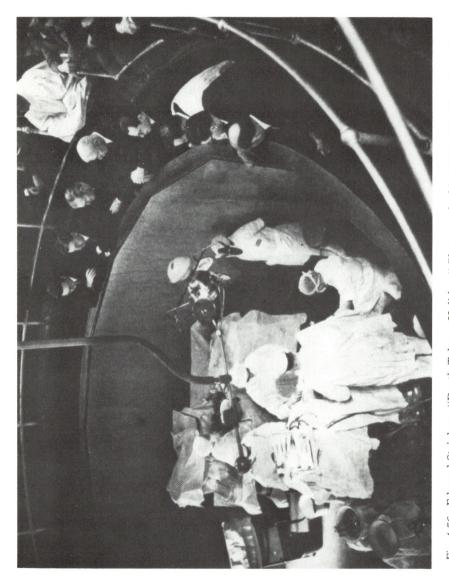

Fig. 4.56 Edward Steichen, "Death Takes a Holiday." Photographed in 1929 at the New York Post-Graduate Hospital for the J. Walter Thompson Agency (Reprinted with the permisson of Joanna L. Steichen).

244

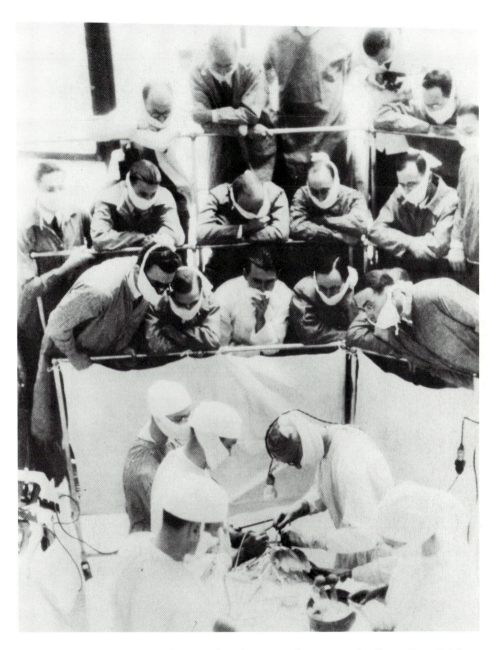

Fig. 4.57 Dr. Harvey Cushing performing a craniotomy at the Peter Bent Brigham Hospital in Boston, 1934 (Countway Library).

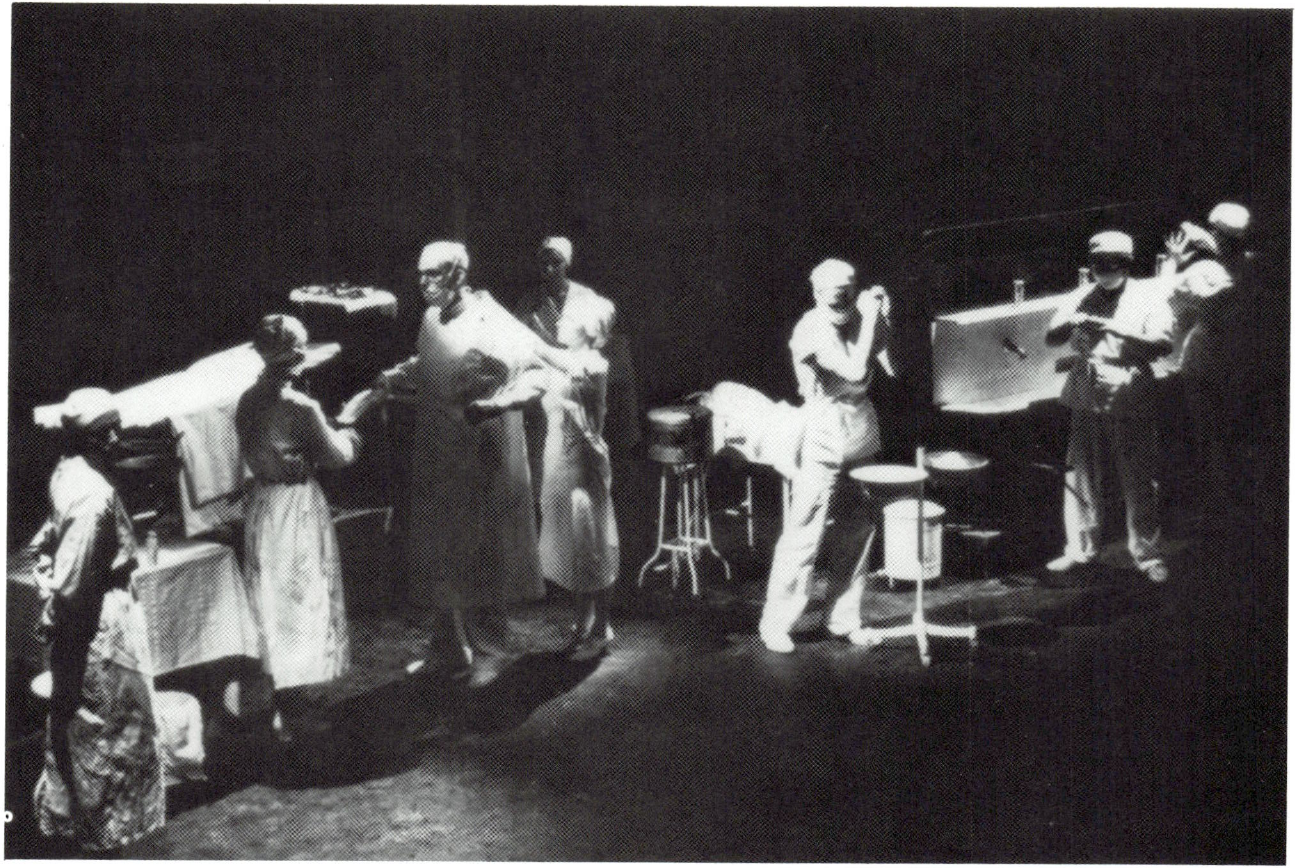

Fig. 4.58 Surgery on the stage set of *Men in White*, 1933 (New York Public Library, Billy Rose Theater Collection).

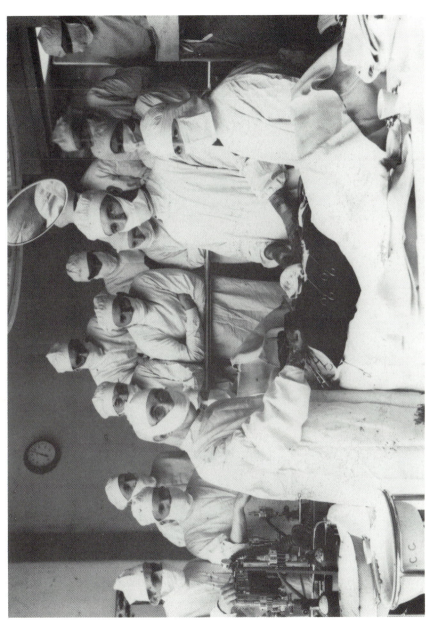

Fig. 4.59 G. Grey-Turner in the operating theatre, Newcastle, March 1940. Although this photograph was probably taken for private use, the picture, characteristically, is close up to the field of operation rather than taking in the whole theatre (Wellcome Institute Library, London).

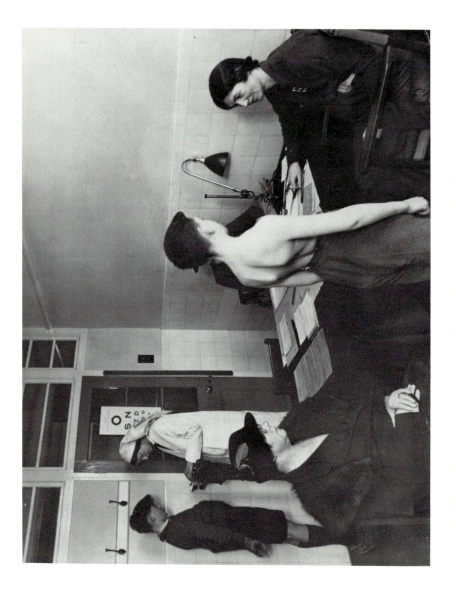

Fig. 4.60 Medical inspection at Avenue School, London, 1938. The depiction of examination in public, in contexts such as this, was still the photographic norm. The obligatory weighing scales were in the background (Greater London Photograph Library—80/5625).

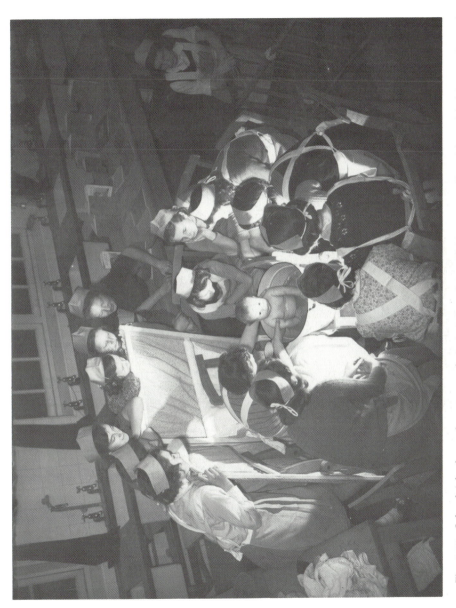

Fig. 4.61 Schoolgirls dressed as nurses learning "mothercraft," purportedly with real babies, at Central School, Lingfield, Surrey, February 10, 1944 (Syndication International [1986] Ltd.).

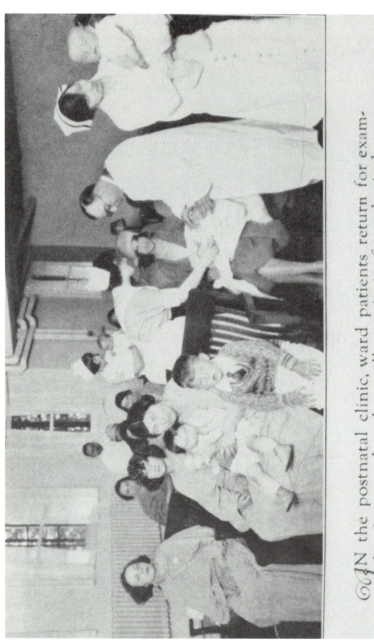

IN the postnatal clinic, ward patients return for examinations so that they will remain in fine physical condition and be guarded against any later complications

Fig. 4.62 Women and Infants Hospital, Providence, Rhode Island, c. 1925 (Women and Infants Hospital of Rhode Island).

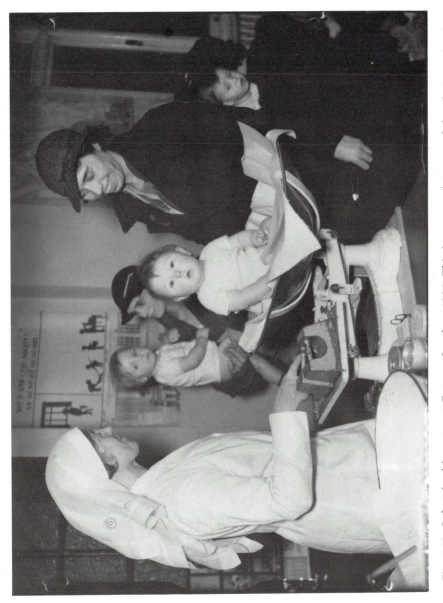

Fig. 4.63 Infant health centre at Putney, London, 1936. This is a press picture, and the photographer has created a close emotional, slightly humorous encounter (Syndication International [1986] Ltd.).

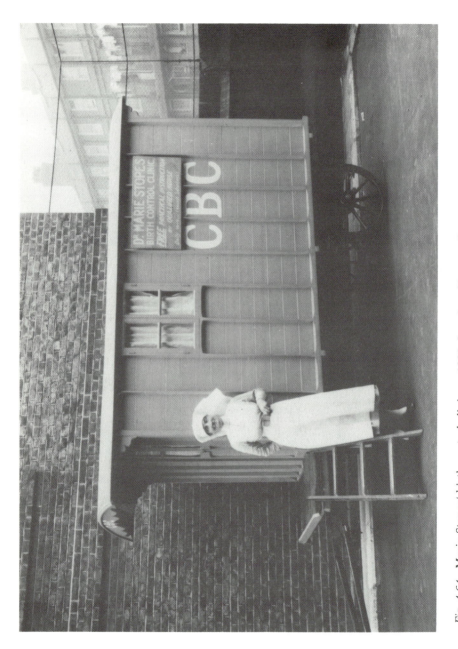

Fig. 4.64 Marie Stopes' birth control clinic, c. 1928. In spite of her conflicts with the medical profession, Stopes depicted her work as medical (Wellcome Institute Library, London).

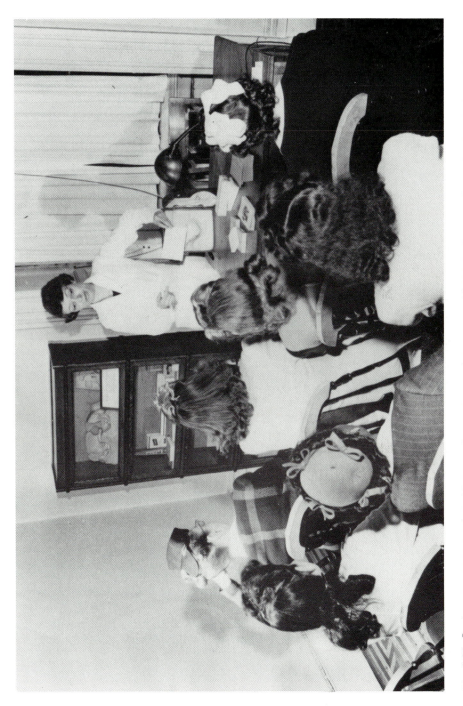

Fig. 4.65 Lecture on contraception, Margaret Sanger Research Bureau, mid-1930s. Compare Fig. 4.64 (Sophia Smith Collection. Smith College).

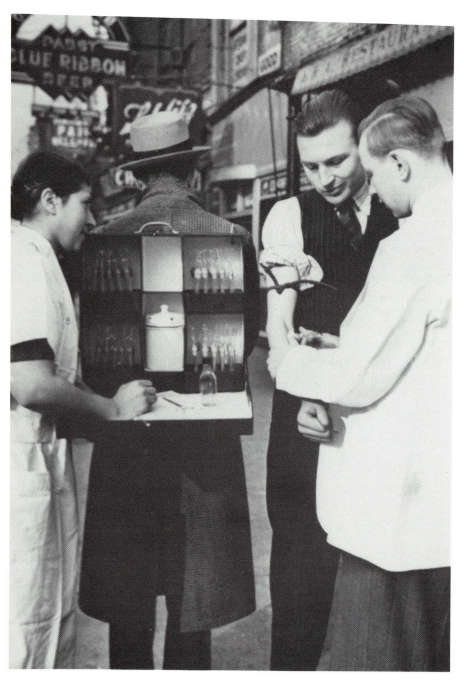

Fig. 4.66 Drawing blood in Chicago, in the late 1930s, under the sponsorship of the federal Works Project Administration (Social Welfare History Archives Center, University of Minnesota).

CHAPTER V

INTENSIFYING THE IMAGE, 1939 AND AFTER

The most obvious characteristic of photographs of medicine taken since the late 1930s is how often the viewer's attention is directed exclusively to the people, particularly the patients, in them. Such photographs gradually, although not entirely, superceded representations of specific interventive measures; diagnostic and therapeutic technology and surgery. To produce these pictures, photographers routinely got closer to people and framed them alone or in small groups. They attended to the facial expressions of their subjects, diminishing the space behind them or making backgrounds indistinct. Press and public relations photographs were cropped to increase the relative size of the people (Fig. 5.1). Wards were no longer represented as spacious and well lit with orderly rows of beds. Everything was excluded from pictures taken in such settings except one or two people and their immediate surroundings (Fig. 5.2). Similarly, surgical photographs were now close-ups of part of a team at work rather than pictures of a whole amphitheater (Fig. 5.3), and photographs of encounters in public health clinics showed only the participants (Fig. 5.4). These photographs, in context, invited viewers to associate medicine with the ideal of attaining a full and healthy life.

This new representation of medicine was the result of changes in photographic style, in the politics of health and in medicine itself. In the 1930s, photographers working in a style called documentary realism had produced detailed studies of the daily lives of ordinary people. When used in journalism, particularly in such magazines as *Life, Look* and *Picture Post*, or in brochures commissioned by hospitals and medical societies, such photographs were made more important than the text, which served mainly to guide readers to see particular messages in the pictures. Medicine was exploited by these photographers as a rich source of personal stories.

At the same time, for other reasons, the individual became more important in medicine. In both countries, access to health services became a political issue. In both, photography was employed to record the provision of health care to individuals and families by government and voluntary agencies. In the United States, and to a lesser extent in Britain, professional medical bodies commissioned photographs from public relations firms. These pictures depicted doctors in close relationships with individual patients.

The taking of photographs in the documentary realist style in medical contexts was also a result of redefinition of the scope of medicine itself. Doctors increasingly asserted responsibility not only for the cure of disease but for total individual health and well-being. From the 1930s onwards there was a growing medical interest in people's everyday lives, in familial and social relationships, and in the social and economic causes of illness. The patient rather than disease was the subject of a new medical literature.[1]

The proliferation of medical photographs in documentary realist style signified public acceptance of medicine's redefinition of its purpose and also public endorsement of its expanding power. By the late 1930s, there was already so much emphasis on the human content of photographs that many pictures no longer represented the institutional setting of medical work. In this photograph from *Picture Post* in 1939, a pregnant woman attended a "pre-natal clinic" which, presumably, was at her local general practitioner's surgery; but it *could* have been at a large hospital outpatient department (Fig. 5.5). Likewise in this picture of a dental patient out of which the photographer and caption writer made a joke, the scene might have been in a hospital or private practice (Fig. 5.6).

When documentary realist photographers did represent hospitals, they were a setting for a personal story. In 1939, for example, *Picture Post* produced five pages of sequential photographs about "A Street Accident and What Follows."[2] Tom Jones, after being hit by a taxi, was rushed to St. Bartholomew's were he was treated for several weeks. Each of the photographs was an intimate portrait of Tom and the skillful people who were caring for him.

Documentary realist photographs of hospital life, although looking different from earlier pictures, still conveyed many of the same norms. This intimate portrait of a nurse and a child (Fig. 5.7) with the mother just visible in the background, when read in the context of the *Picture Post* story "Visiting Day" in which it appeared, reinforced the hospital's requirement that the families of patients abnegate all authority and responsibility to its staff. Similarly, *Picture Post*'s jocular account of the "Nurses' Ball" used stereotypes of medicine and nursing. The nurses laughed and "enjoyed themselves" while the picture and text combined to suggest that doctors were serious people (Fig. 5.8).

Some medical situations were not yet photographed as human interest stories. In pictures dealing with cancer, possibly because the disease was so generally regarded as fatal, new therapeutic technology, not the patient, was usually the subject (Fig. 5.9). *Life*, for example, in 1938 published a photo-essay which described a "War on Cancer" primarily by representing scientific apparatus.[3] Visual imagery of personal struggle against this disease was not yet as acceptable as it was in the case of, say, tuberculosis and, from the late 1930s, among people who had suffered poliomyelitis and who were undergoing rehabilitation.

Documentary realist photography was extensively employed during the Second World War. The war was represented by government and the press in both countries as a heroic struggle by ordinary people, and many members of the public apparently concurred. The comradeship that was stimulated by wartime events, at home and abroad, was a frequent subject for popular dramatization in photographs as well as in other media. For military reasons too the individual fighting man had become a subject of greater concern than in earlier wars.[4]

Two pictures taken at the beginning of the war exemplify the use of both older and newer styles of photography. The first is an official photograph of a British officer examining a Maltese recruit (Fig. 5.10). It is a close-up of two people. But the photograph was composed with a spacious public background much as it might have been twenty years earlier. The second photograph, of an American recruit being immunized, was taken for *Life* by George Strock (Fig. 5.11). At first, it appears to be almost the same representation as the previous photograph. Both depict the sacrifice of the privacy of the medical encounter in the public interest. But *Life*'s readers, who were familiar with the visual language of photojournalism, could have given Stock's composition several additional meanings; for example, about American individualism, the bravery of the common man, and, not least, the power of scientific medicine directed to preserving the *public* health.

Wartime medical photographs frequently depicted doctors or other personnel with patients at close range (Fig. 5.12). Unlike American photographs of this time, British pictures still carried messages about class. In this close-up, a pipe and a cricket sweater were reminders that the doctor was a gentleman at war (Fig. 5.13).

During the First World War, trained women had frequently been photographed caring for wounded soldiers. In the Second World War, photographers took such pictures at closer range and paid particular attention to facial expressions (Figs. 5.14, 5.15). Also for the first time, male medical personnel were occasionally photographed in intimate caring relations with the wounded (5.16).

Blood transfusion was one of the most frequent subjects of war photography. Numerous close-up pictures were taken of wounded soldiers receiving blood (Fig. 5.17). People at home knew that tranfusion was an extraordinarily successful procedure for preventing shock (Figs. 5.18, 5.19). Photography displayed the use of this relatively simple technology which was based on sophisticated science (Fig. 5.20). These pictures also celebrated and cemented the gift relationship between the soldier abroad, receiving the blood, and those giving it at home.

American war photographers frequently represented wounded soldiers rehabilitated by medicine. Such pictures were used to publicize medical success and personal readjustment. To a victorious nation they signalled that, as a result of medicine, men who had sacrificed for their country were now restored to civilian life (Fig. 5.21).

The homefront was a particularly important subject for British photographers because it was also a theater of war. *Picture Post* and other publications used photographs to support morale and to endorse the government's management of the war. These photographs, their captions, and the accompanying text presented to the British public an image of itself as patriotic, democratic, activist, resilient and, above all, cheerful (Fig. 5.22).[5] Photographs representing the recovery of individuals from illness as a result of collective action may also have been read as showing the necessity for teamwork in order to win the war (Fig. 5.23). Dozens of the most ordinary pictures taken in medical settings depicted people apparently accepting waiting and discomfort in good humor (Fig. 5.24). Photographs of busy outpatient departments were probably now used to signal community sacrifice for the war effort, in addition to the older message that ordinary people must accept waiting and public treatment as appropriate for their class (Fig. 5.25).

After the war, the human interest photographic style that was standard in the press was increasingly used for official pictures of hospitals, clinics, and other medical settings. Images that were once associated only with the hospital began to appear in quite different contexts (Fig. 5.26). The construction of pictures that combine personal concern and medical expertise and appear to be "slices of life" requires considerable craft. Less skillful photographers sometimes were not wholly successful in the creation of such images (Fig. 5.27).

When we discussed hospital imagery in Chapters III and IV, we drew attention to its domestic and later its industrial resonances. Photographers who depicted hospital interiors after the war showed them as workplaces for efficiently managed scientific teams delivering personal care. The new model was modern business. No single picture demonstrates this. The new imagery can only be appreciated by examining the variety of photographs that hospitals employed in reports or promotional literature. Such publications presented all departments of a hospital, especially the technical ones, as parts of an integrated system which delivered personal care.

In photographs promoting the message that hospitals offered attention to individuals, images of crowded clinics were no longer appropriate. This photograph from a hospital brochure showed just one person arriving for an outpatient appointment (Fig. 5.28). Because it was used to convey a meaning so obviously at variance with people's continuing experience of waiting in crowded outpatient departments in both countries, this photograph exemplifies our insistence that representations cannot be used as privileged sources for the documentation of health care, past or present. Like other sources they are rhetorical accounts that require interpretation.

By the 1950s, the organization of hospitals was becoming increasingly complex and power within them fragmented among different branches of the medical profession. Photography, in turn, was part of the making of these emerging medical specialities, just as it had been part of the making of surgery fifty years earlier. This is a photograph of an American anesthesiologist in 1950 (Fig. 5.29). Such pictures were unusual before this time. Photographers of surgical operations before the Second World War rarely portrayed anesthetists but, as their professional status grew in the 1940s, pictures of them became more frequent outside their own journals. This photograph of an anesthesiologist, published in a popular health magazine, was not a surgeon's image of the operating theatre. It was an image of the anesthesiologist's work made by using the conventions of photojournalism to depict, in a corner of the room, the man, the machines, and the head of the patient. Photographers also represented hospital teams, emphasizing their human as well as their technical face. This picture of a cardiac care team in Liverpool depicted *ordinary* individuals working together to deliver personal care through science and technology (Fig. 5.30).

The new power of medical scientists after the war can also be studied in photographs. Laboratory research as a source of progress was now extensively depicted by photojournalists, supplementing, and to some extent replacing, the images of technology that stood for science in earlier photographs (Figs. 5.31, 5.32).[6]

The increasing uniformity of photographs of general hospitals was accompanied by the disappearance of the distinctive image of special hospitals. This is hardly surprising, since in these years general hospitals in both countries were caring for increasing numbers of patients with chronic and contagious conditions that had previously been the responsibility of special institutions. Even asylums increasingly appeared as places where patients received physical, pharmacological or surgical therapy. This picture of ECT or shock therapy resembles other contemporary images of nurses overseeing medical treatment (Fig. 5.33). Moreover, psychoanalysis in hospital settings was represented as in-depth personal *medical* therapy. The editor of *Picture Post* placed this photograph alongside a picture of psycho-surgery (Fig. 5.34).

In these years, for the first time, images were published that were critical of custodial care in the absence of medical intervention. Photojournalists produced human interest stories about the plight of patients in the back wards of hospitals for the mentally ill or disabled. *Picture Post*'s famous photograph taken "behind the farthest locked door" in an asylum was meant, according to the accompanying text, to depict patients who were, at present, beyond the reach of therapy (Fig. 5.35). American photographs of patients in the back wards helped to create an imagery of the "snake pit" which leading psychiatrists used to justify their advocacy of institutional reform (Fig. 5.36).[7]

Nurses have remained an immensely popular subject with photographers. Since the First World War, they have appeared in diverse and sometimes inconsistent images. Most frequently they were depicted as skilled, hard working, dedicated people with a vocation (Fig. 5.37). Often the photographs represented them as caring for, as well as taking care of, patients. (See Fig. 5.61 for this distinction). Photography has largely ignored male nurses. It has been used to present an image of nurses as women, whose femininity was defined by impeccable grooming, interest in babies, fashion and sexual awareness (Figs. 5.38, 5.39).[8] These photographs of nurses were particular perceptions, just as earlier representations had been.[9] The conventions for photographing nurses were quite distinct from those employed to depict women doctors (see Fig. 5.49) who were represented as professionals and only incidentally as women.

This diverse imagery of nurses was part of an expanding definition of the scope of medicine. In the 1930s, for the first time, photographs represented pre-natal care. This photograph depicted a group of pregnant women being instructed in the biology of reproduction by a woman in a white coat (Fig. 5.40). It advertised that part of the responsibility of local government in the provision of maternity services was the transmission of medical knowledge. In both countries, photographs of childbirth were published in national magazines, where it was depicted as a medical event. In 1946 *Picture Post* published a photo-essay about the delivery of a baby at home. A picture taken soon after birth exemplifies the skill of a first-rate human interest photographer (Fig. 5.41). The baby dominated the photograph, framed between the midwife's hands and its mother's thighs. The white sheet and towel and the basin signalled the security provided by medicine in a domestic delivery. Similarly, a subsequent photograph in the series showed a masked and gowned midwife weighing the baby. Versions of this image soon appeared in more mundane contexts (Fig. 5.42).[10]

The publication of photographs of childbirth in America began with stills from the controversial hospital film "The Birth of a Baby" which appeared in *Life* shortly before the war.[11] These photographs, like those taken in Britain, represented childbirth as a time when medical interest legitimately extended beyond technical expertise to include the involvement of doctors and nurses in family life. In Britain, the midwife was shown introducing siblings to the newborn (Fig. 5.43). Similarly, an American nurse introduced a father to his child in a hospital nursery (Fig. 5.44).

A famous series of human interest photographs about the work of a midwife was taken for *Life* by H. Eugene Smith in 1951. These photographs are striking because of Smith's extraordinary use of light and his mastery of dramatic composition (Fig. 5.45). The mother is entirely absent from this photograph.

From the late 1930s, close-ups of babies and children in medical photographs were taken at their own level, thus increasing their relative prominence in the picture. (Compare with the photographs in Chapter III.) A wartime close-up illustrates the use of this convention to depict a familiar subject—weighing the baby (Fig. 5.46).[12]

The candid photograph was a device frequently used in these years to depict medical encounters as pleasant experiences for children and families (Fig. 5.47). In many photographs children smiled, even when the picture represented what are usually considered painful or uncomfortable procedures—an inoculation or physical examination, for example (Fig. 5.48). Here is a British photograph of a smiling doctor immunizing a baby while its mother and a cut-out parrot looked on (Fig. 5.49). It appears candid, but the procedure could have lasted only a moment and the photographer took at least one other picture of it, this time including Pinnochio (Fig. 5.50).

In Chapters III and IV we noted that before the 1930s, photographs of mothers and children often represented them as deferring to medical authority. (See, for example, Fig. 3.111.) Such deference was not represented in postwar pictures (Fig. 5.47, for example), not because it was absent from *actual* encounters but because of the redefinition of medicine as a vocation caring for individual needs, not as an institution necessary for dealing with the sick poor. For example, in this photograph of a mother showing off her baby at a fertility clinic, the mother and baby have been made the center of the picture. The nurses are represented simply as admiring young women (Fig. 5.51).

After the war, patients were only rarely depicted in public settings with other people near them. In this close-up of a screening program for venereal disease in New York in the early 1950s, an encounter involving a stigmatizing disease was photographed as a public event (Fig. 5.52). Another exception was the picture of a doctor at the Windmill theater in London, inoculating chorus girls against influenza. No doubt it was taken to demonstrate that the theater lived up to its slogan—"We never closed" (Fig. 5.53). The similarity in the composition of this photograph and George Strock's picture of a soldier being inoculated (Fig. 5.11) suggests that people in certain occupations were assumed to have no right to privacy.

Photographs of consultations between doctor and patient have remained rare. A few photographs of medical encounters were used by hospitals and professional associations for distinct political ends. A photograph taken in 1948, for a magazine published by the American Medical Association, was the self-image of one of the factions in American medicine (Fig. 5.54). In the late 1940s, a so-called "grass roots movement" in the American Medical Association championed what it claimed was the intimate personal approach of the family doctor against the indifference of the specialist and the increasing absorption of doctors in hospital work.

Similarly, in 1955, the Middlesex Hospital in London produced a brochure describing its work in text and photographs. It is evidence for the convergence of American and British visual imagery of the ideal medical encounter that the hospital chose for its cover a photograph which was almost identical in composition to the previous picture (Fig. 5.55). Some of the meanings that viewers were invited to associate with this extremely complex photograph were reinforced by other pictures in the booklet. This initial image of skillful human care would have been seen in the context of subsequent photographs that displayed impersonal, effective, scientific therapy. Thus in a later photograph surgery was anonymous and mechanical and the patient was not represented at all (Fig. 5.56). The booklet also included a story about Patrick, a young man who, like Tom in the *Picture Post* story of 1939, was knocked down in the street. The story represented the events of Patrick's hospital stay in precisely the same visual language employed by *Picture Post* sixteen years earlier.

On the rare occasions when general practice in either country was photographed after the war it too was represented through multiple complementary images. These photographs almost invariably represented doctors who practiced in rural areas. The pictures were strong statements—and, when they are viewed in the context of other sources, political statements—about how general practitioners perceived themselves. The photographs declared that these doctors valued their intimate knowledge of their patients and their technical skill and resented the encroachment of specialists and hospitals on their practices.[13]

In 1948, *Life* published a remarkable photo-essay by Eugene Smith entitled "Country Doctor." Smith represented his doctor as scientifically trained and maintaining a personal interest in his patients. Smith's skill endowed this doctor with more attributes than other doctors previously presented in photographs (Figs. 5.57, 5.58, 5.59). The text that accompanied the photographs encouraged the reader to see rural general practice as both noble and frustrating.

British photographs of general practice carried similar messages. In the early 1950s, a British photographer, guided by two general practitioners, produced a sequence of pictures about rural practice called "Country Doctor." It was used to teach schoolchildren as one of a series, "Men at Work." The photographs, which represented the doctor at his daily work in his surgery and on home visits, were, like Eugene Smith's pictures, a normative account of general practice (Fig. 5.60).[14] According to this account, general practitioners should properly take responsibility for the physical and psychological well-being of an entire community. Doctors should do this without regard to their own rest or convenience. In 1967, another British general practitioner was depicted as *A Fortunate Man* by John Berger and Jean Mohr in a book subtitled *The Story of a Country Doctor*.[15] Mohr used the same conventions as the other documentary realist photographers did to depict skillful, responsible doctors. Not surprisingly, therefore, despite Berger's sensitive text about the doctor's personal life, the book endorsed, as most medical photographs have done, doctors' perceptions of themselves and their power.

Several years later, Berger declared that as a result of the inevitable ambiguity of photographic images, photo-stories must depend on words.[16] Most historians have not heeded Berger's warning. Rather, they have shared the familiar epistemological assumption that photographs unambiguously reveal the past. The unquestioning use of this assumption necessarily leads historians to behave as though photographs are objective statements.

The photographs in this book could have been used to tell a familiar story about the history of medicine. Our text, however, tells a rather different story. It is a story about how images were made and used to carry messages. These were messages about how and where medical power should be exercised and by whom. Subsequent historians will surely quarrel with our story, in whole or in part. That is the fate of most historical works. We will, however, regard it as an achievement if historians challenge our method in order to extend their understanding of the epistemological problems of the photograph.

In the months before this book went to press several new images of medicine appeared. This is not surprising; new images are continually being made as perceptions of the role of medicine change. One of the most important sources of these new perceptions is medical power itself. A picture which appeared in an English newspaper in January 1987 is not like most other representations of medicine during the last fifty years (Fig. 5.61). The figures are distorted and stand apart, a great deal of space is included, the beds are bare. It is not a close-up. It is not a human interest picture. An imagery for AIDS is being made.

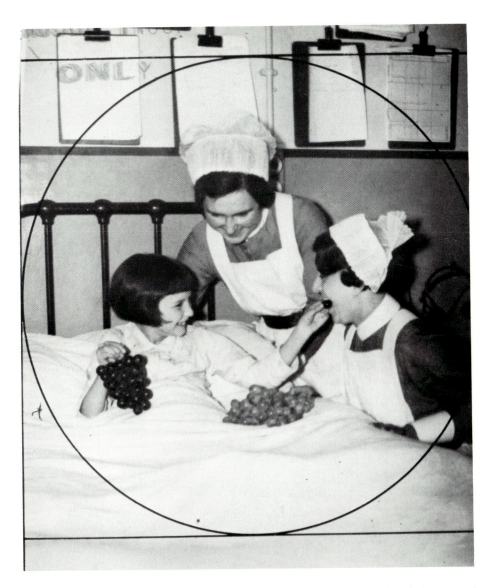

Fig. 5.1 A post-war press photograph from the Westminster Hospital, n.d. A note on the reverse says 'Grapes from St. James's Palace,' The Westminster hospital was particularly proud of its connection with Royalty; this child presumably had just received a royal present of grapes. The editor circled the area of interest and the final print was to be the square enclosing the diameter of the circle (Riverside Health Authority).

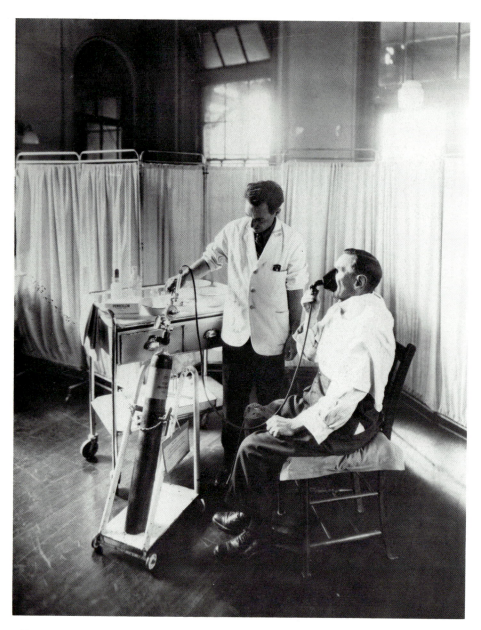

Fig. 5.2 Assistant nurse, St. John's Hospital, London, 1947. The unusual feature in this photograph is the depiction of a male nurse. Pictures of female nurses seem to outnumber those of male nurses disproportionately to their ratio in the profession (Greater London Photograph Library—80/7400).

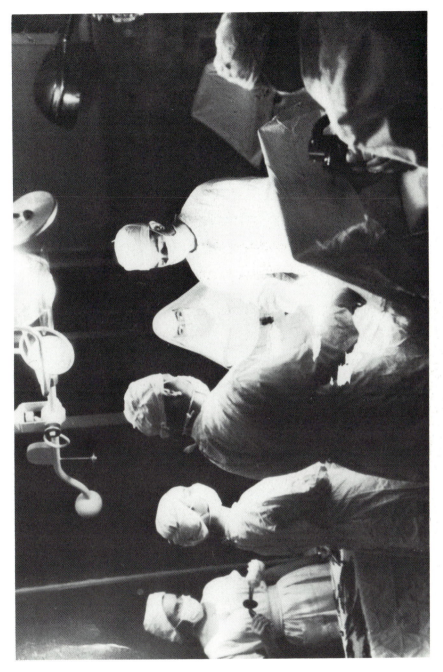

Fig. 5.3 Surgery at St. Joseph's Hospital, Atlanta, Georgia, in the early 1950s (St. Joseph's Hospital, Atlanta, Georgia).

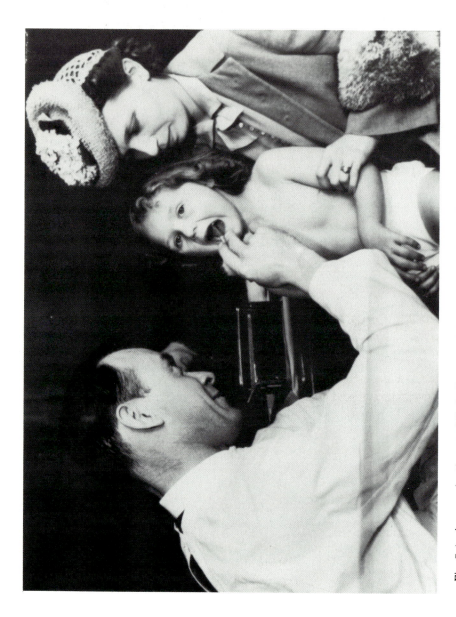

Fig. 5.4 An examination at a Works Progress Administration clinic in Lake Wisconsin in 1939 (State Historical Society of Wisconsin—c. file 82).

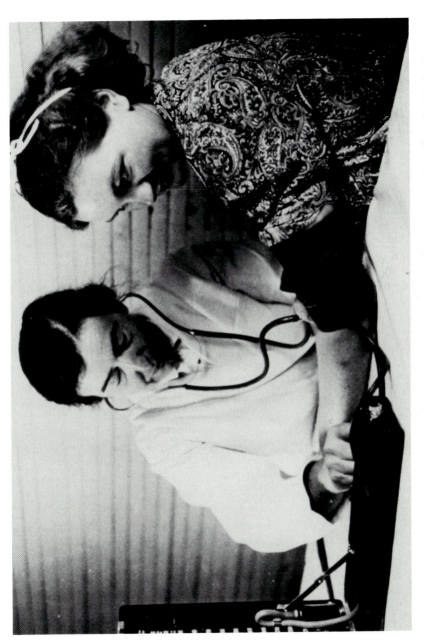

Fig. 5.5 From the *Picture Post* story, "A baby is born at home." The caption read "Before the birth: the doctor checks up" and indicated that the picture was of a weekly visit to a "pre-natal" clinic. *Picture Post*, August 31, 1946, p. 8 (BBC, Hulton Picture Library).

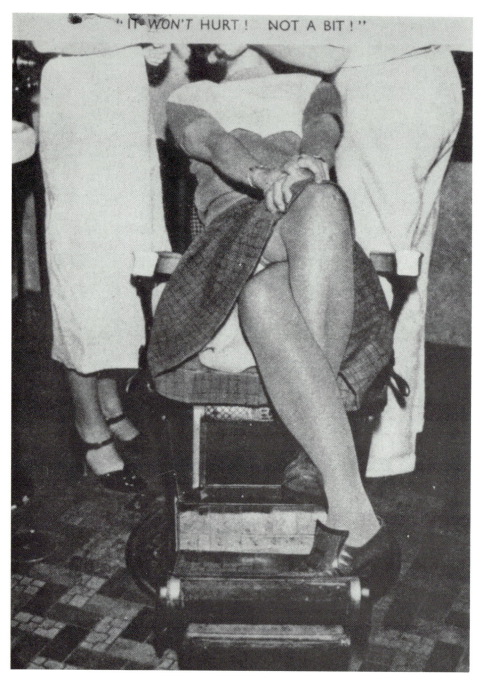

Fig. 5.6 A *Picture Post* photograph accompanying a humorous verse about the dentist's chair. *Picture Post*, January 14, 1939, p. 61 (Owner unknown).

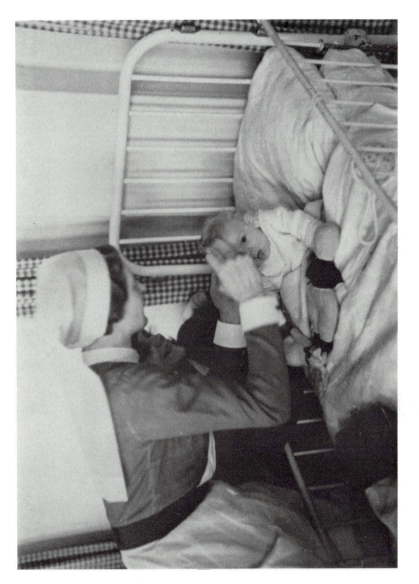

Fig. 5.7 From a *Picture Post* story, "Visiting day." A typical *Picture Post* photojournalistic report of an ordinary event, one of the two weekly afternoons on which St. Bartholomew's allowed its patients to have visitors. The nurse bestowed attention on the child while the mother was almost obscured. The caption also explained that the baby's older sister was not allowed a visit since she was not yet fourteen. *Picture Post*, March 11, 1939, p. 53 (BBC, Hulton Picture Library).

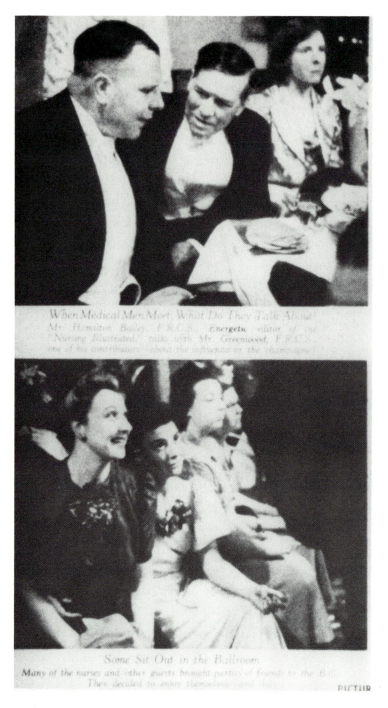

Fig. 5.8 From a photostory, "Nurses ball," *Picture Post*, April 15, 1939, p. 46. Compare the similar depiction in Fig. 4.32 (BBC, Hulton Picture Library).

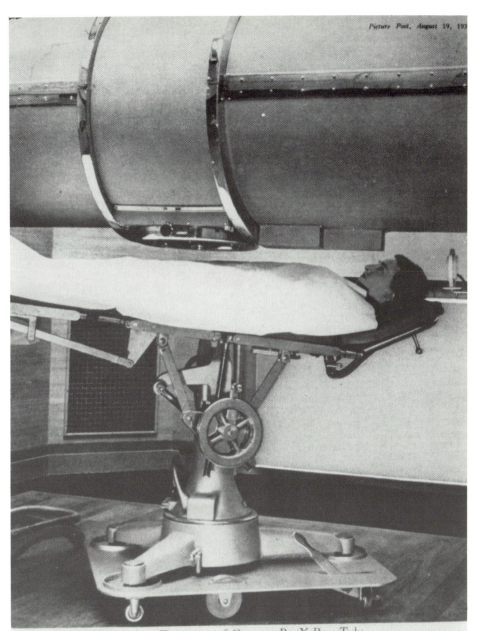

The Modern Treatment of Cancer: By X-Ray Tube

The X-ray tube in position with the patient beneath it. The walls round are radiation proof: no one can be in the same room for fear of damage. For six hours a day cancer is bombarded thus. St. Bartholomew's Hospital cannot afford to maintain beds for the patients who might be saved if the tube could be used for twenty-four hours in the day.

Fig. 5.9 From *Picture Post*: "Cancer," a story describing "the present stage in our struggle to conquer man's most terrifying enemy." Although endeavoring to be optimistic about the future diagnosis and management of cancer, the article painted quite a bleak picture, noting particularly that X-ray therapy was "difficult and dangerous." *Picture Post*, August 19, 1939, pp. 60-62 (BBC, Hulton Picture Library).

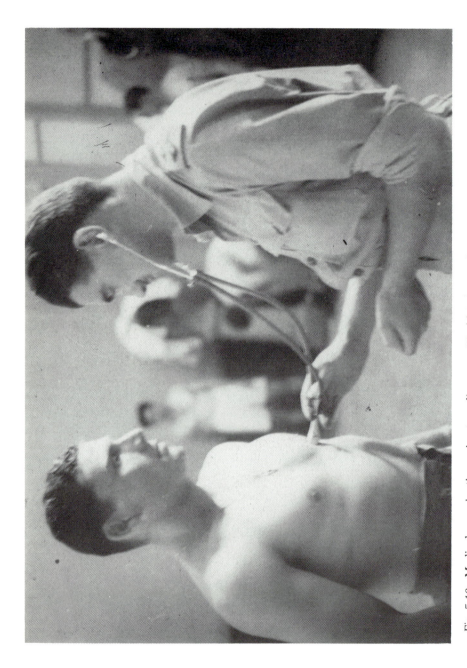

Fig. 5.10 Medical examination prior to enlistment. World War II (The Trustees of the Imperial War Museum, London—NA3912).

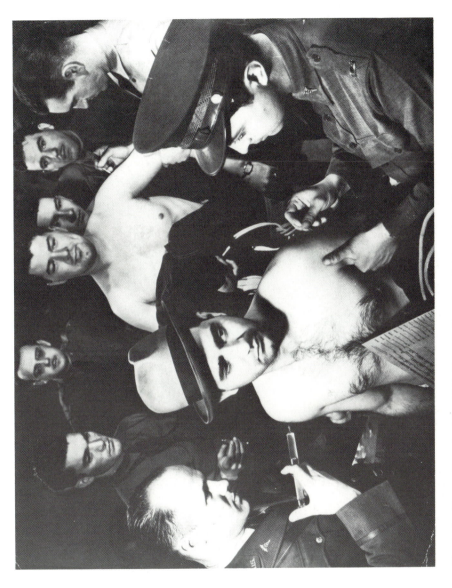

Fig. 5.11 George Strock, *Life*, 1941 (George Strock, *Life* Magazine, © Time Inc.).

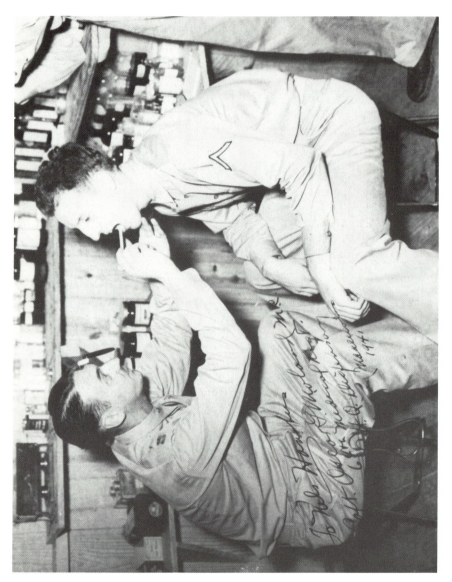

Fig. 5.12 Doctor and patient at General Headquarters Dispensary, Louisiana (Luther Hospital, Eau Claire, Wisconsin).

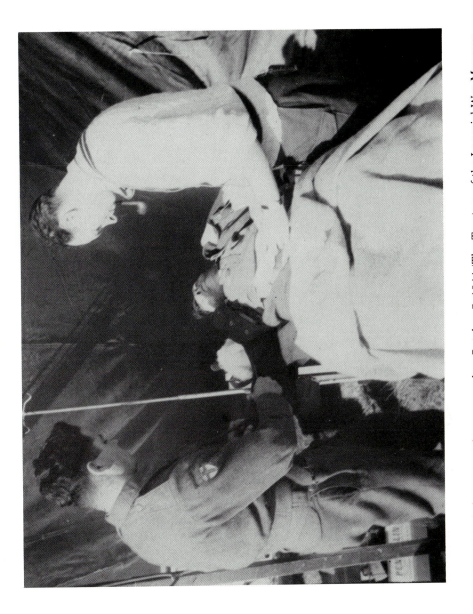

Fig. 5.13 A doctor examines a casualty, October 5, 1944 (The Trustees of the Imperial War Museum, London—B10549).

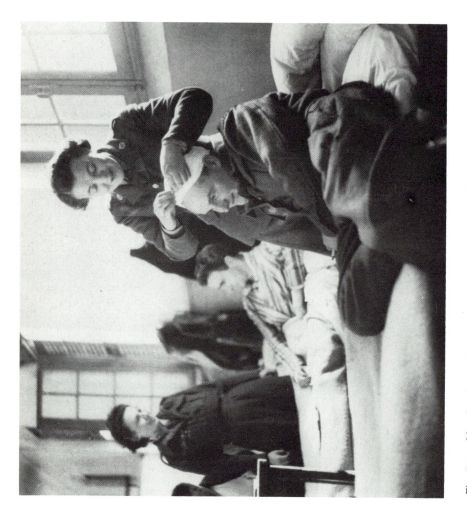

Fig. 5.14 Nursing Sister dressing a wound at the 94th Field General Hospital, February 1, 1943 (The Trustees of the Imperial War Museum, London—NA794).

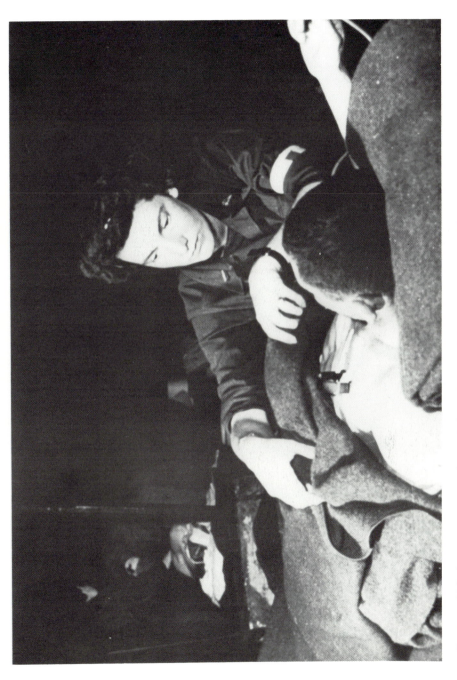

Fig. 5.15 U.S. Army nurse caring for a soldier with a lung injury, France, 1944 (Methodist Hospital, Madison, Wisconsin).

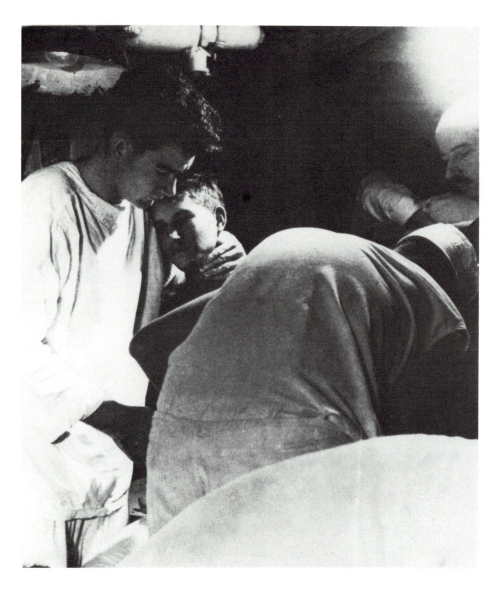

Fig. 5.16 Attendant and soldier, aboard U.S.S. *Solace*, near Okinawa, 1945 (National Archives of the United States—Department of the Navy—80-G-413963).

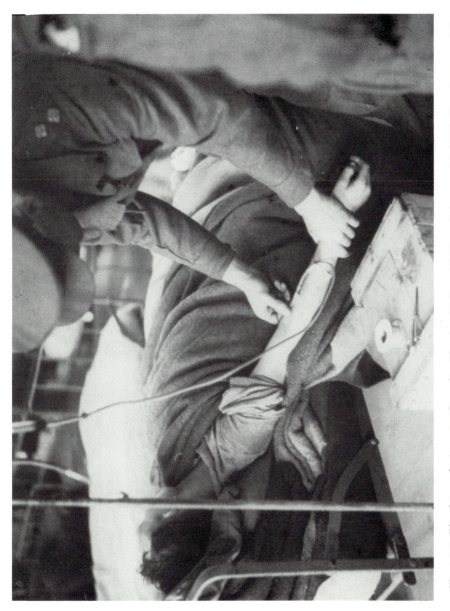

Fig. 5.17 Blood transfusion at a Casualty Clearing Station, Thirbar, February 11, 1943 (The Trustees of the Imperial War Museum, London—NA715).

281

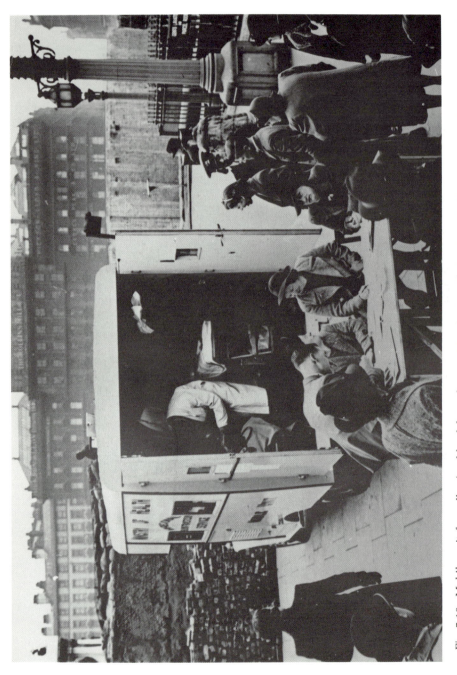

Fig. 5.18 Mobile unit for collecting blood from donors. Manchester, England, 1941 (Manchester Public Libraries: Local History Library).

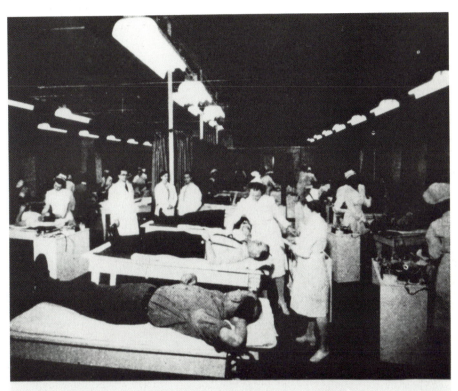

The bleeding room accommodates 39 donors at one time. The foot end of each table is raised 5 inches to ensure high venous pressure.

Fig. 5.19 Donating blood, Boston, Massachusetts, 1943 (*Modern Hospital*, 1943, now *Modern HealthCare*, © Crain Communication, Chicago, Illinois).

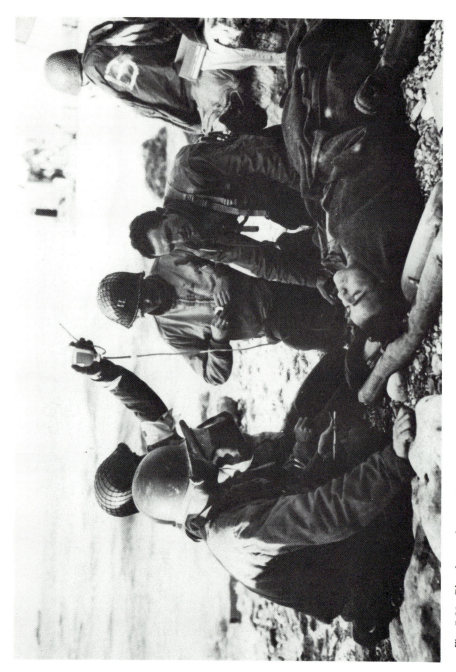

Fig. 5.20 Blood transfusion during the invasion of Normandy, 1944 (American Red Cross, Washington, D.C.).

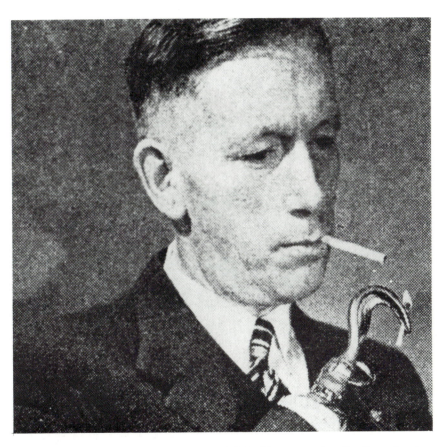

Fig. 5.21 This 1944 photograph was published in a magazine distributed to the general public by the American Medical Association (*Hygeia*, 1944, 22:422).

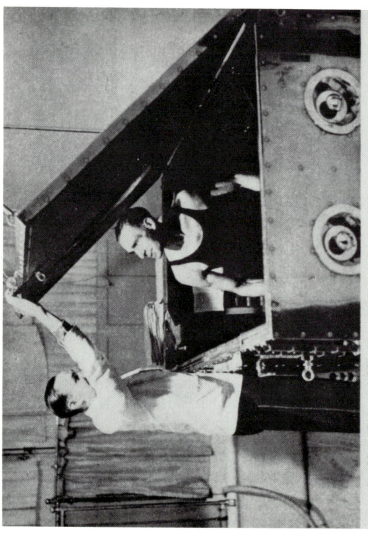

"In You Go, and You Don't Come Out Till You Feel Better!"

It's a thermal vapour bath. There'll be a big demand for it when Tommies have experienced their first Winter at the Front. You sit inside the cabinet, head out of the top **21**

Fig. 5.22 From a *Picture Post* photostory, "Bath awaits the wounded" which described how the springs at Bath were being used in the treatment of men from the Front. *Picture Post*, January 13, 1940, p. 21 (BBC, Hulton Picture Library).

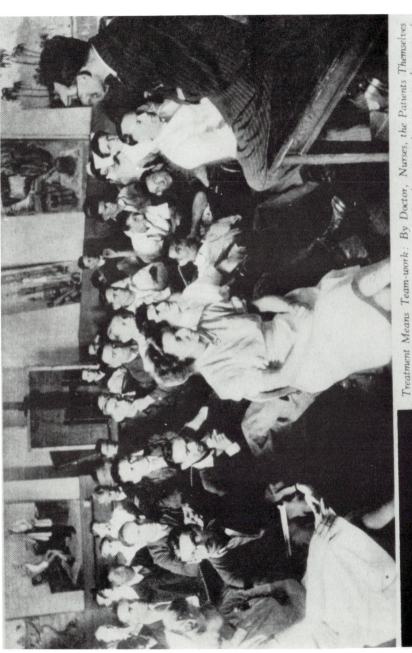

Treatment Means Team-work: By Doctor, Nurses, the Patients Themselves
One of the principles of neurosis treatment is that the patient takes part in it. In a series of group talks, the doctor discusses nervous troubles frankly. Nurses join in, too.

Fig. 5.23   From the photostory, "A hospital for war nerves." *Picture Post,* July 22, 1944, p. 11 (Owner unknown).

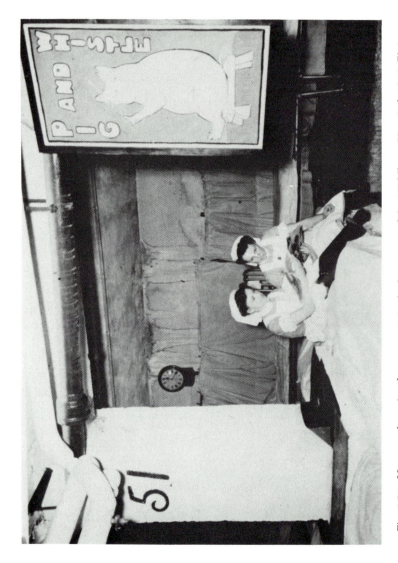

Fig. 5.24 Nurses rehearsing for a concert in the basement of the Middlesex Hospital, 1940. Pictures of hospital doctors relaxing are rare (The Archivist of the Middlesex Hospital).

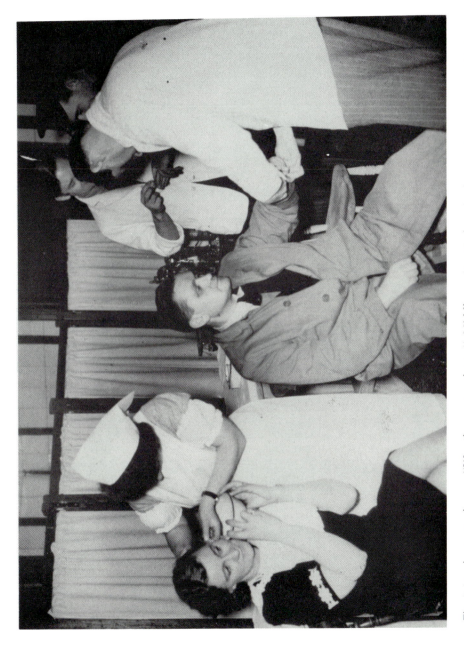

Fix. 5.25 A press picture "War-time outpatients," Middlesex Hospital, n.d. (The Archivist of the Middlesex Hospital).

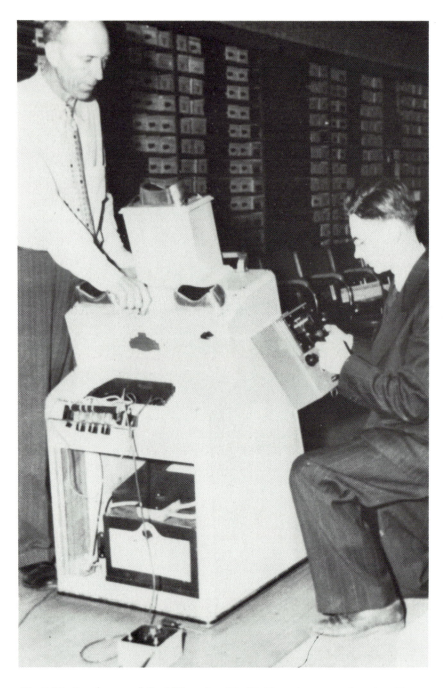

Fig. 5.26 Employees of the Milwaukee Health Department testing shoe X-ray machine in a department store, 1950 (City of Milwaukee, Health Department).

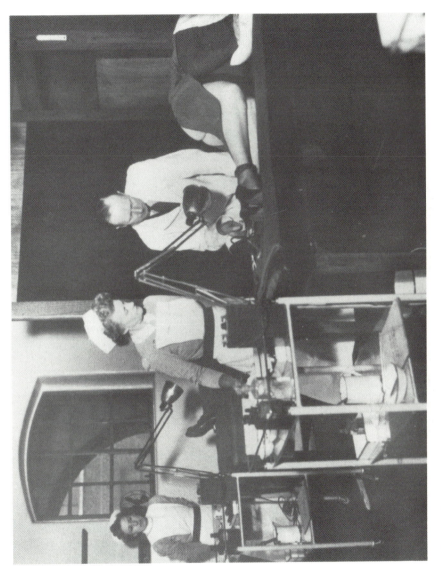

Fig. 5.27 Outpatient Department, St. Mark's Hospital, London. The photographer evidently intended to combine personal care and technology into the usual sort of composition, but the angle chosen and the amount of background produced a slightly odd effect (St. Mark's Hospital, London).

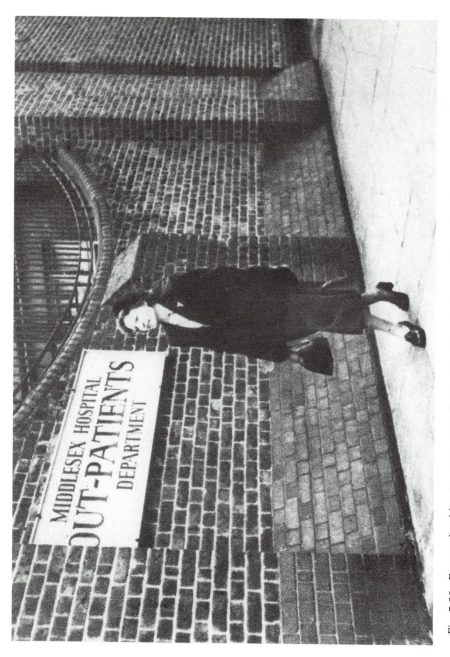

Fig. 5.28 From a booklet *Hospital at Work* (London: The Middlesex Hospital, 1954), advertising the hospital (The Archivist of the Middlesex Hospital).

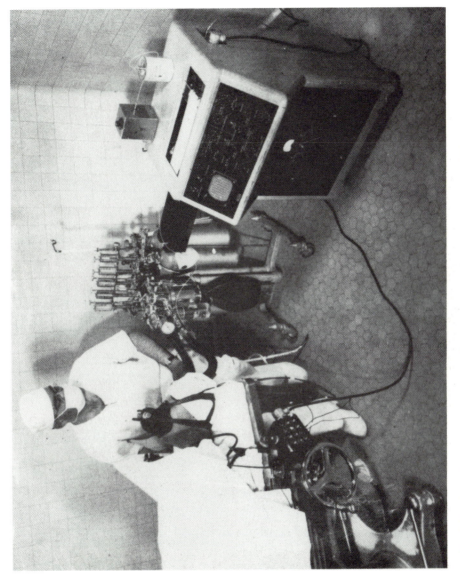

Fig. 5.29 Anesthesiologist at work, 1950 (*Today's Health*, 28: September, 1950).

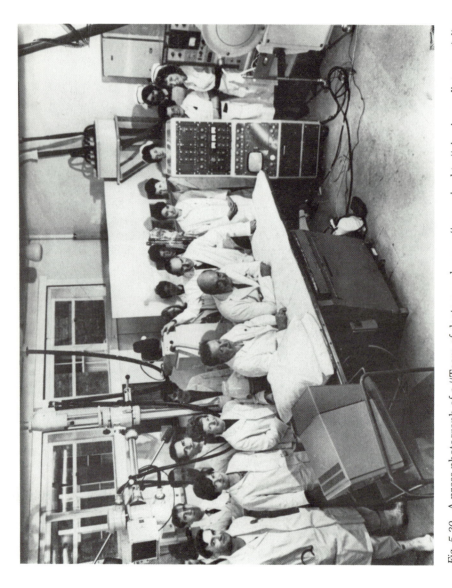

Fig. 5.30 A press photograph of a "Team of doctors and nurses" organized to "give immediate specialist attention to serious heart attack cases," n.d. (*Daily Herald* Picture Collection, copyright unknown).

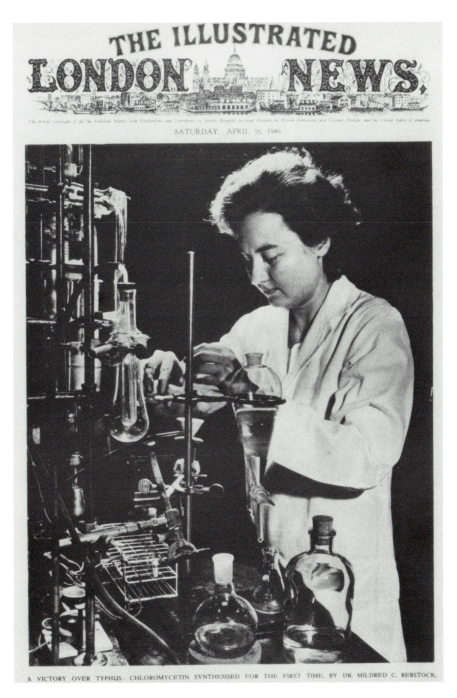

THE ILLUSTRATED LONDON NEWS,

SATURDAY, APRIL 16, 1949.

A VICTORY OVER TYPHUS: CHLOROMYCETIN SYNTHESISED FOR THE FIRST TIME, BY DR. MILDRED C. REBSTOCK.

Fig. 5.31 Front cover of *The Illustrated London News,* April 16, 1949. This must have been the photojournalist's dream picture: a woman, a doctor, medical research and a wonder drug (*The Illustrated London News* Picture Library).

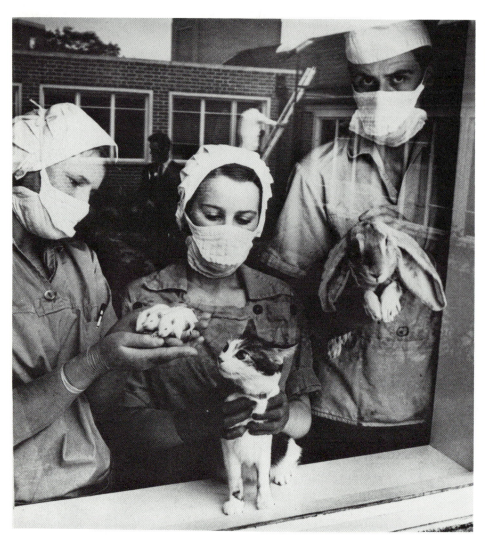

Fig. 5.32 A press photograph of the Medical Research Centre, Carshalton, 1968. This picture combined human and animal interest with medical progress. Subsequent anti-vivisectionist activity might have encouraged other readings of such pictures which would now be unacceptable to newspaper editors (Syndication International [1986] Ltd.).

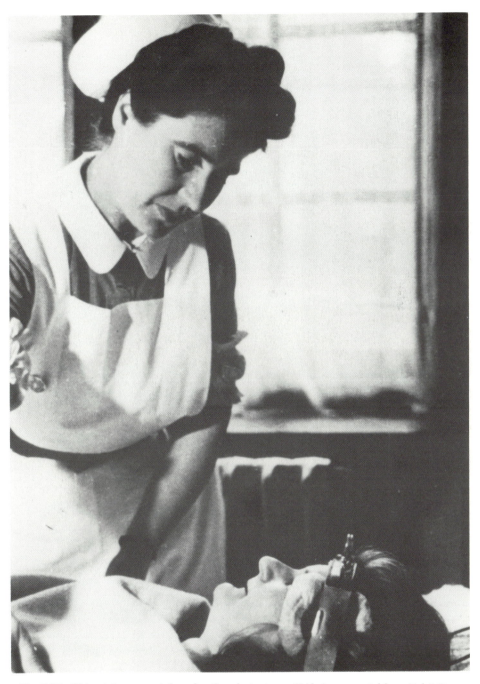

Fig. 5.33 This picture was taken for the photostory, ''Life in a mental hospital.'' It was not used, but a similar image was published, depicting two nurses. It was entitled, ''she is jolted out of hell.'' *Picture Post*, November 23, 1946, p. 12 (BBC, Hulton Picture Library).

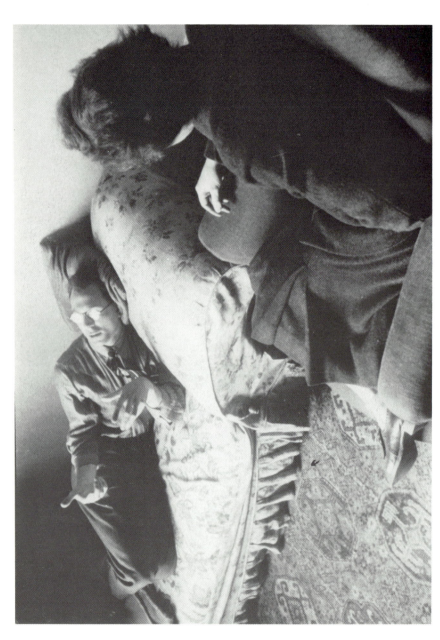

Fig. 5.34 From the same article as Fig. 5.33, entitled "The subconscious is probed," p. 13. The possibility of finding a photograph representing a medical encounter in this way twenty years earlier seems remote (BBC, Hulton Picture Library).

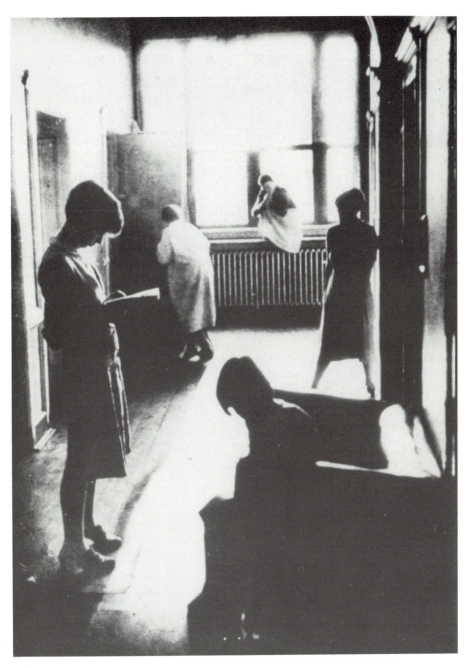

Fig. 5.35 From the same article as Fig. 5.33, entitled "Behind the farthest locked door where there is little hope." The text noted "The woman attitudinizing on the right used to go about naked; the brain operation known as leucotomy has so far composed her that she dresses now" (BBC, Hulton Picture Library).

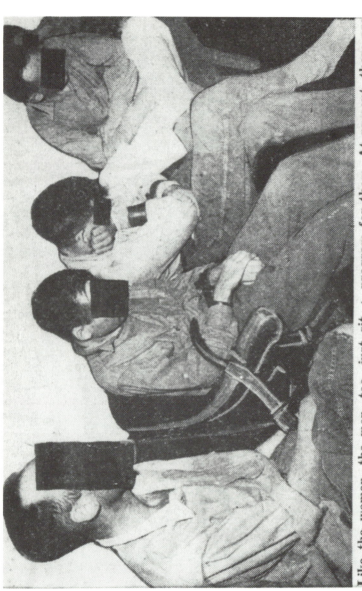

Like the women, the men, too, just sit shackled to each other or to the chairs. This wouldn't be the case if the hospital had enough help to provide a recreational program for them. At present, there are six nurses and six doctors taking care of the patients which is far below the number needed.

Fig. 5.36 A Wisconsin newspaper account of the results of insufficient medical staffing, 1947 (Mendota Mental Health Institute, Madison, Wisconsin, scrapbook of newspaper articles).

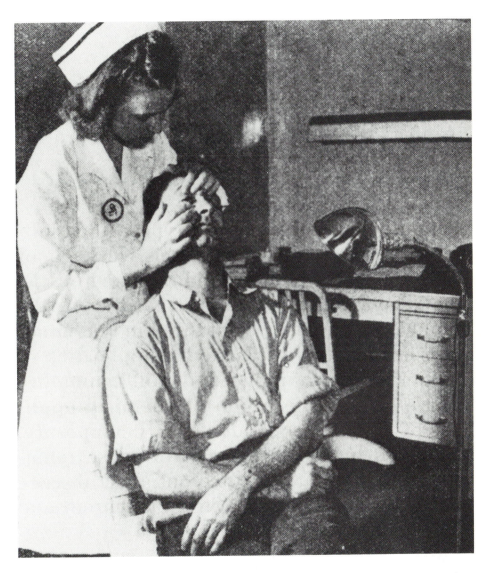

Fig. 5.37 Nurse treating a worker with an injured eye, Boeing Company war plant, Wichita, Kansas, 1945 (*Hygeia*, 1945, 23:194).

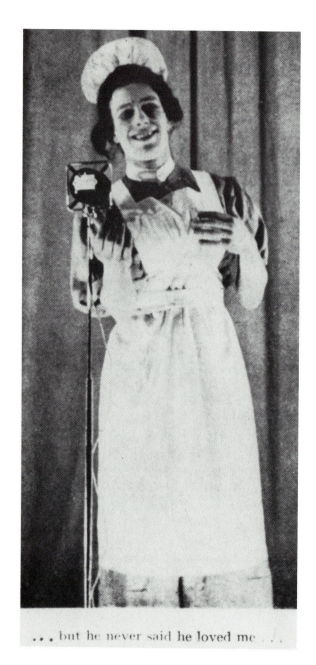

. . . but he never said he loved me . . .

Fig. 5.38 A medical student in the Christmas show at the London Hospital, 1946. It is not simply that nurses became objects of parody after the war, they may have been that before; rather, it became an acceptable activity which photography legitimated and showed how it might be done (*London Hospital Gazette*, 1947, *50*:facing p. 6).

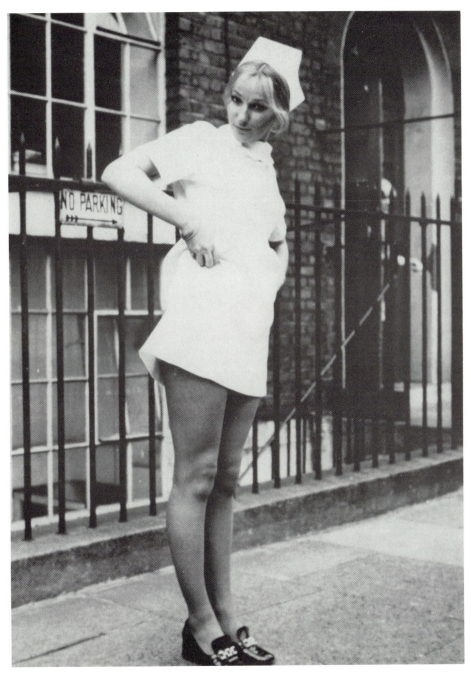

Fig. 5.39 Press photograph of a model wearing a new uniform for nurses, London, 1969 (Syndication International [1986] ltd.).

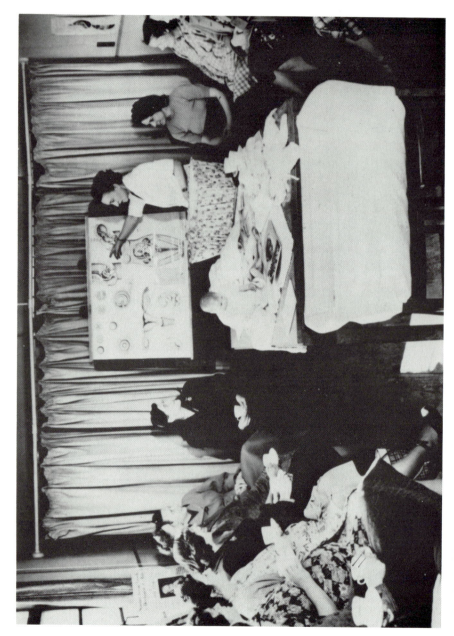

Fig. 5.40 The maternity Welfare Centre, Harrow Road, Paddington, London, c. 1950 (Greater London Photograph Library—80/7364).

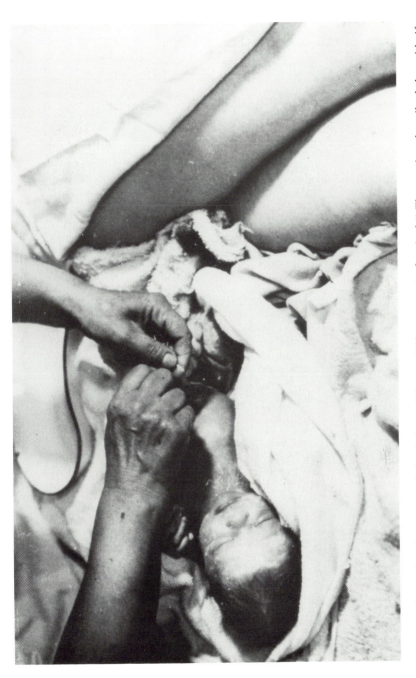

Fig. 5.41 From the photostory a baby is born at home, "The moment of arrival." The caption described the midwife tying the cord in the front bedroom of a five-room council house in Kent. For a few years, until hospitalization of delivery occurred, this was the image many British parents had of what their baby's birth ought to be like. *Picture Post*, August 31, 1946, p. 8 (BBC, Hulton Picture Library).

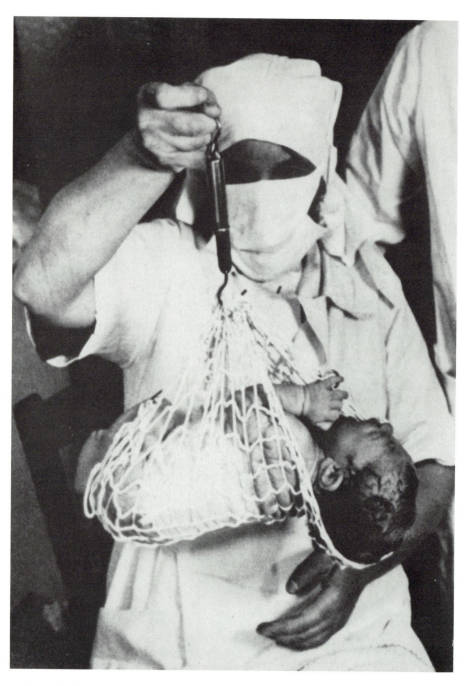

Fig. 5.42 From the same story as Fig. 5.41, entitled "The verdict." Note the old theme—weighing the baby—dramatically depicted (BBC, Hulton Picture Library).

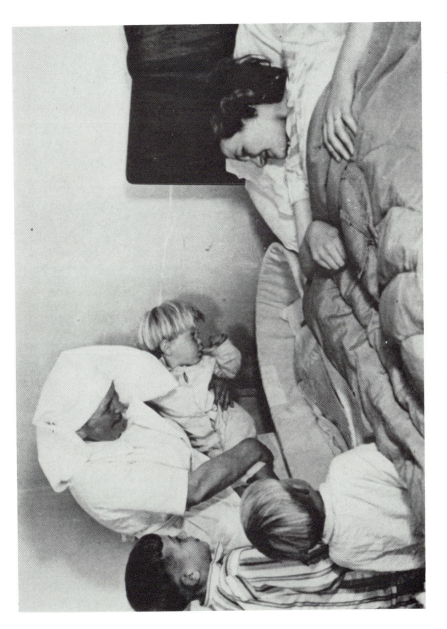

Fig. 5.43 From the same story as Fig. 5.42, entitled "Janet is introduced to her brothers." The father never appeared in any picture, nor in the story, where reference was made to the "whole family" (BBC, Hulton Picture Library).

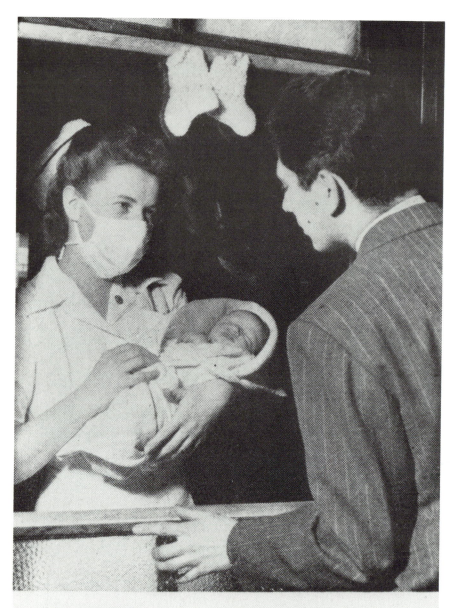

A proud if weary Dad catches his first glimpse of his new daughter—through glass.

Fig. 5.44 This photograph was published in a magazine distributed in doctors' offices by the American Medical Association. Presumably it was used to teach fathers their role in childbirth (*Hygeia*, 1948, 26:109).

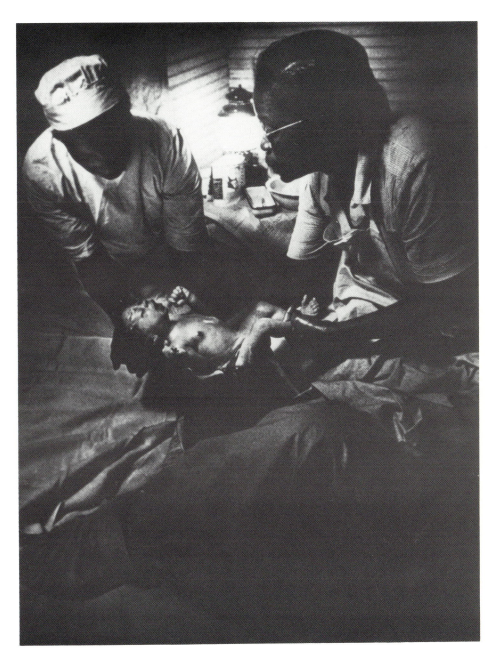

Fig. 5.45 Nurse-midwife Maude Callen and her assistant hold a newborn a few minutes after birth; Pineville, South Carolina, 1951 (W. Eugene Smith: Black Star).

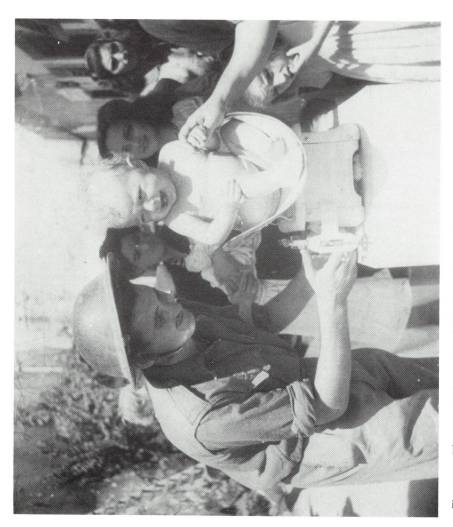

Fig. 5.46 The Royal Army Medical Corps in Sicily, World War II (The Trustees of the Imperial War Museum, London—NA5562).

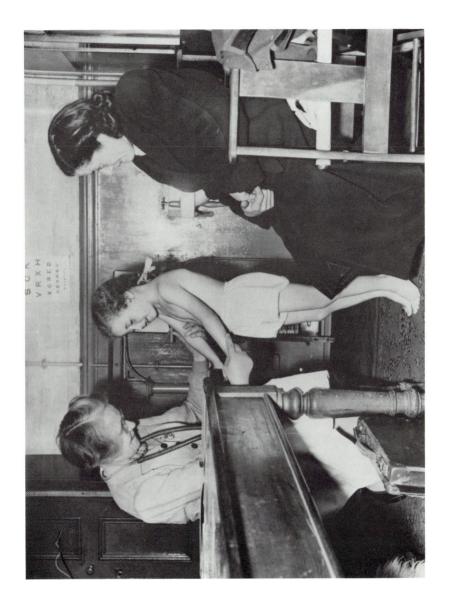

Fig. 5.47 Medical inspection, Belleville School, Wandsworth, London, 1949 (Greater London Photograph Library—80/3628).

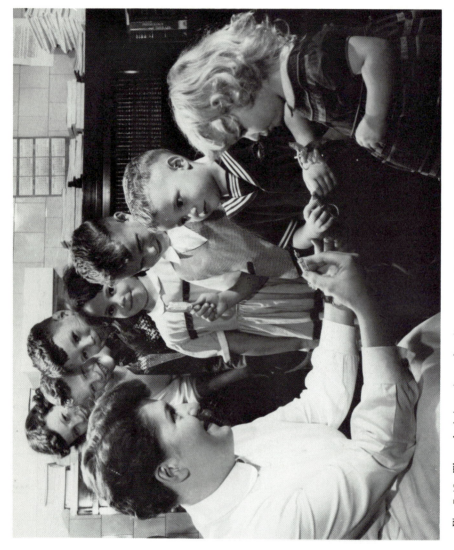

Fig. 5.48 The administration of polio vaccine in Milwaukee, Wisconsin, 1955 (State Historical Society of Wisconsin—c. file 4166).

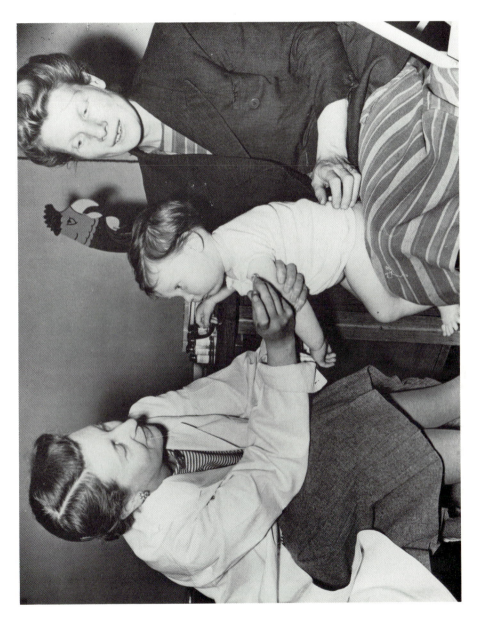

Fig. 5.49 Hackney Clinic, 1949 (Greater London Photograph Library—81/9345).

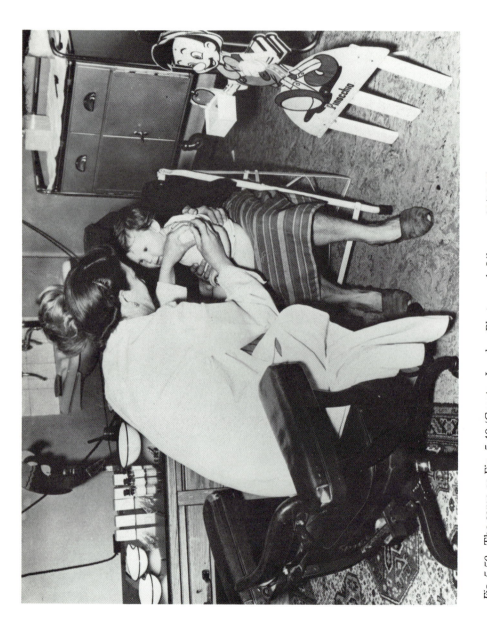

Fig. 5.50 The same as Fig. 5.49 (Greater London Photograph Library—81/9347).

314

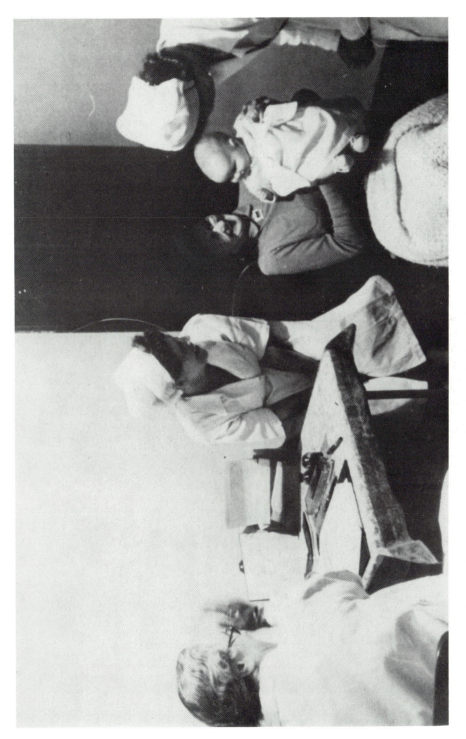

Fig. 5.51 A family planning clinic, n.d. (BBC, Hulton Picture Library—M1930).

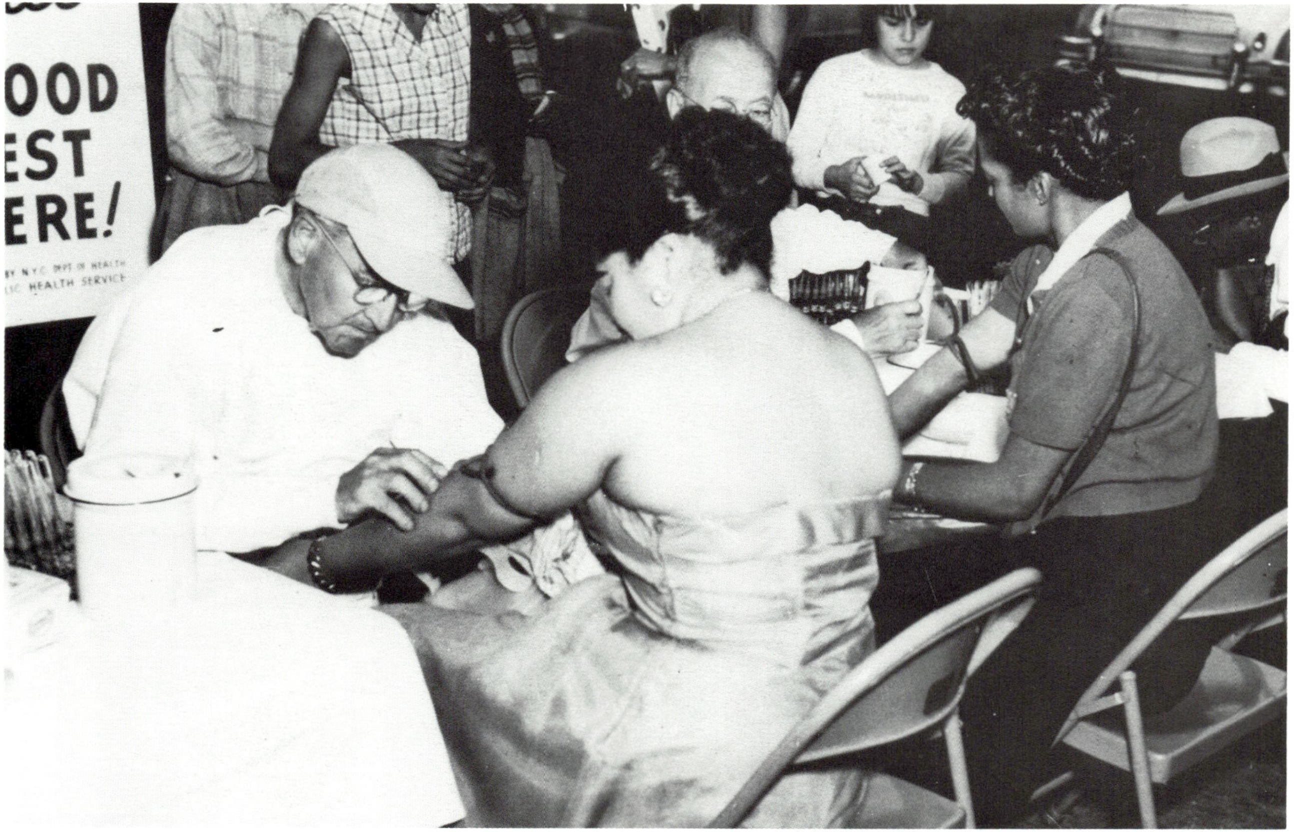

Fig. 5.52 Testing for venereal disease in New York City, 1953 (Social Welfare Archive, University of Minnesota).

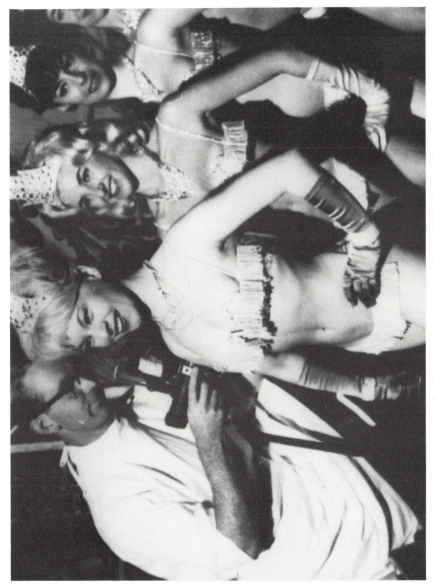

Fig. 5.53   One of a series of press photographs of Windmill Girls, 1963 (Syndication Internation [1986] Ltd.).

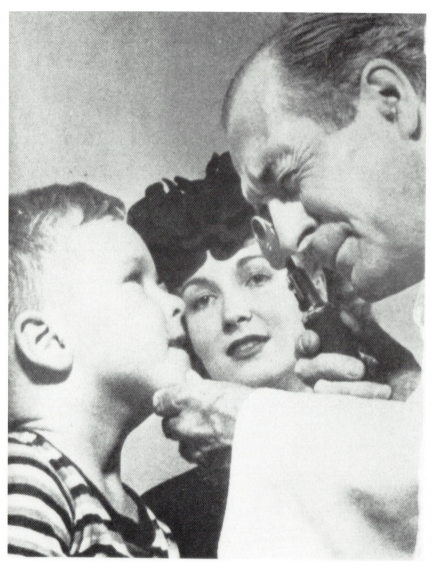

Fig. 5.54 Like Fig. 5.44, this photograph was commissioned by the American Medical Association (*Hygeia*, 1948, 26:268).

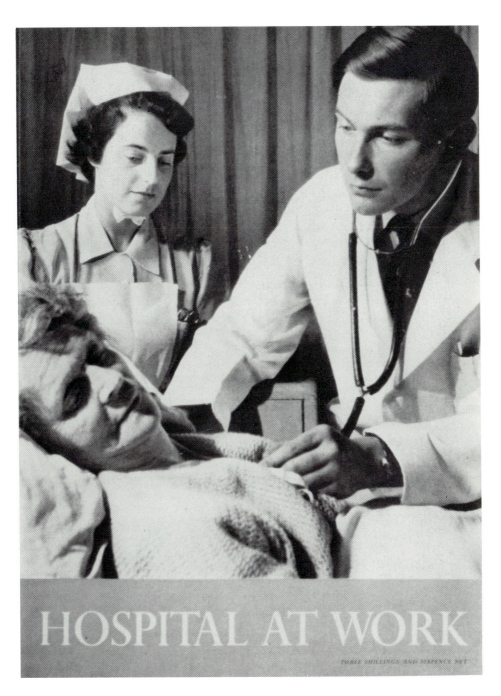

Fig. 5.55 Front cover of *Hospital at Work* (London: The Middlesex Hospital, 1954. The Archivist of the Middlesex Hospital.)

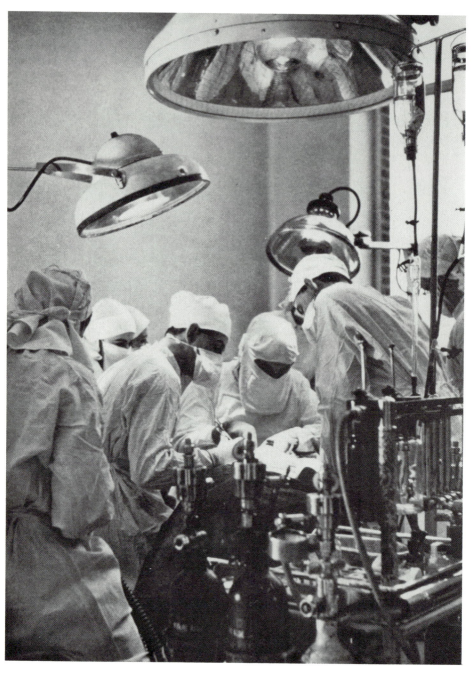

Fig. 5.56 From the same source as Fig. 5.55 entitled "The Thoracic Surgeon Operates," p. 43 (The Archivist of the Middlesex Hospital).

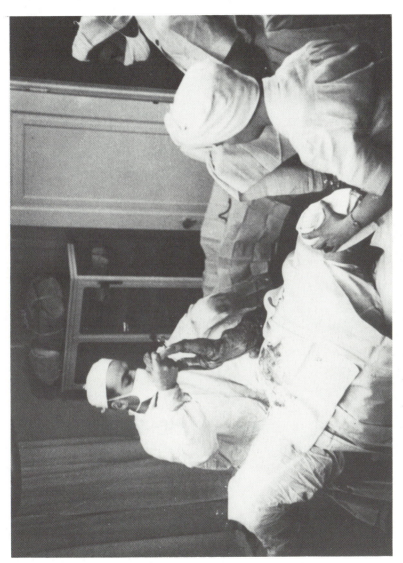

Fig. 5.57–5.59 This photograph, and Figs. 5.58 and 5.59, were part of the photo essay "Country Doctor" by W. Eugene Smith, published in *Life* in 1948. Smith's photographs, frequently published and exhibited, have been discussed as part of the history of modern photography; they also belong to the history of medical images (5.57, 5.58, 5.59, W. Eugene Smith: Black Star).

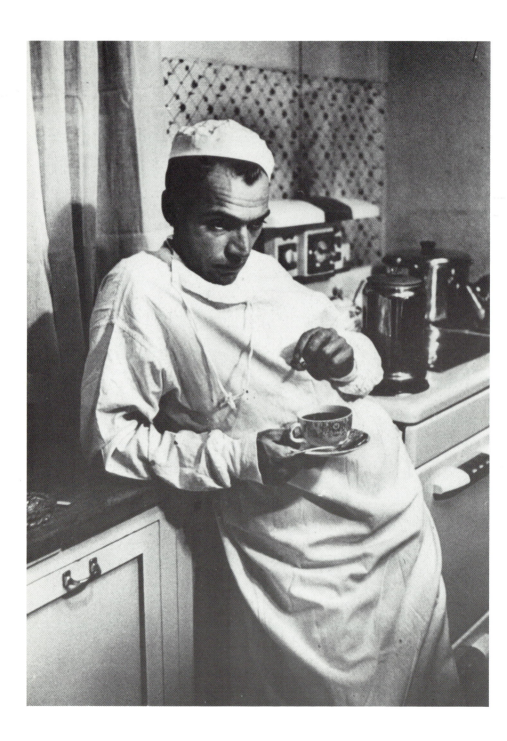

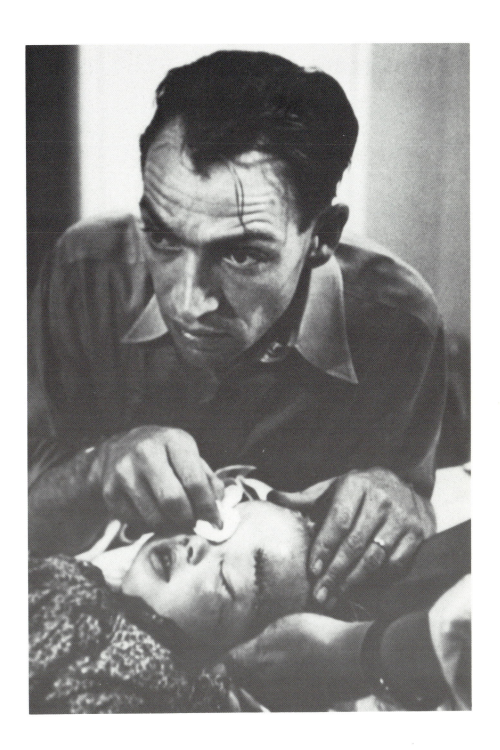

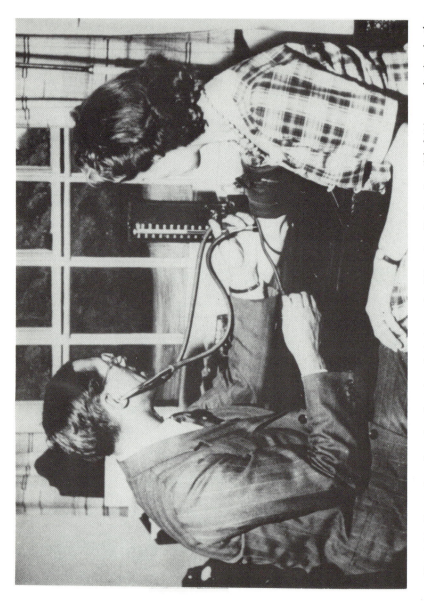

Fig. 5.60 From the educational series of photographs "Country Doctor," entitled "A consultation in the surgery." Stephen Hadfield *Country Doctor* (London, Common Ground Ltd., 1950) (Courtesy of Dr. S. Hadfield and Dr. C. Barber).

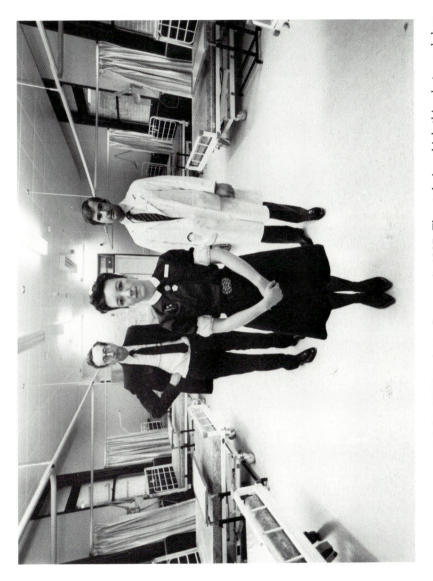

Fig. 5.61 A new ward for AIDS patients, January 9, 1987. The style in which this photograph has been made is not unique—it can be found in pictures of the police and of the inhabitants of run-down areas in towns, for example (*The Independent*, Friday, January 9, 1987, Herbie Knott).

SOURCES FOR THE HISTORY OF MEDICINE AND THE PHOTOGRAPH

MEDICAL PHOTOGRAPHS

The photographs in this volume were selected after extensive research in books and periodicals, public archives and private collections, in Britain and the United States. Many thousands of medical photographs survive. These exist in various states of preservation. There has unfortunately been a general lack of interest by historians, institutions and archivists in preserving photographs. In general, survival in a good state of preservation has usually depended on individual initiatives and enthusiasms. Conversely, simple survival is often a result of lack of interest in clearing out old files. Early clinical material is often well preserved in medical photography departments. Other photographs usually fare less well, except in institutions which pride themselves on their past.

There is a convenient guide to American medical photographs, the *Illustrated Catalogue of the Slide Archive of Historical Medical Photographs at Stony Brook* (Westport, Conn.: Greenwood Press, 1984). The catalogue describes and indexes 3,171 photographs selected as representative of those in American archives and publications. It lists archival and institutional sources, selected books and articles containing significant historical medical photographs and explains how slides can be obtained at cost from the archive. Most of the American photographs in this book were included in the catalogue.

There is no comparable British publication. The following account of British sources is not intended to be exhaustive. It is simply a general guide to the sorts of archives which contain photographs and an indication of the best specific sources. Although there is no British guide to medical photographs there is John Wall, *Directory of British Photographic Collections* (London: Heinemann, 1977). This guide, however, contains a number of errors and often fails to distinguish between historical material and modern working libraries of clinical and pathological photographs. There is a useful guide to picture libraries, Rosemary Eakins, ed., *Picture Sources U.K.* (London: Macdonald, 1985), but references to medical material may mean only engravings, etchings

and other handmade prints. There are four particularly fine photographic collections in Britain which contain a great deal of medical
material. None of them have published catalogues, yet all are relatively
well sorted and accessible. These are the Greater London Photograph
Library, the Beamish Open Air Museum, the Manchester Studies Unit of
Manchester Polytechnic, and the Library of the Wellcome Institute for
the History of Medicine. The Imperial War Museum has a well cata-
logued, specialized collection of photographs pertaining to both World
Wars which contains many medical pictures. The Royal Photographic
Society Library at Bath has been inaccessible and is indexed only by
photographer. Communications with the staff suggest that the medical
content is negligible. Newspaper and periodical libraries are variable as
sources, but invaluable are *The Illustrated London News* Picture Library
and The BBC Hulton Picture Library, the latter containing the remarkable
Picture Post collection. A particularly fine source is the *Daily Herald*
Picture Library. This is now housed at the National Museum of
Photography, Film and Television at Bradford. Unfortunately the
photographic collections of most national daily newspapers are
inaccessible directly, because they have been destroyed, or are not
systematically preserved, or access is only permitted through picture
agencies. Of these agencies, Syndication International holds a great deal
of media material, especially relating to the *Daily Mirror*, but most of the
photographs are post-Second World War. This is not only because of the
holding policy of the agency but also because relatively little medical
material appeared in print before 1940.

After these major sources, the historian has to turn to local institutions.
Hospitals are the obvious candidates, and in many of these there are
collections in various states of preservation. Three of the finest London
hospital collections are at St. Bartholomew's, the Middlesex, and the
Westminster. In the provinces, Birmingham General Hospital holds two
large photographic albums, and the Edinburgh Royal Infirmary has a
substantial collection. Leeds Infirmary has a small, relatively inaccessible collection. Most asylums have small collections but one of the best
preserved and finest is at the "Sunnyside Asylum" in Montrose. Friern
Barnet, surprisingly, has very few pictures. The Royal College of
Psychiatrists has a reasonable but uncatalogued collection. The other
London Royal Colleges—Physicians, Surgeons, Obstetricians, Nursing,
and General Practitioners—have only collections of portraits. Local
authorities are extremely variable in their holdings. The Greater
Glasgow Health Board has an excellent, well preserved collection of
photographs containing a great deal of medical material. Local libraries,
for instance Manchester and Leeds, very often contain medical material
and persistence may be rewarded since such material often may not be
classified as medical. After exploring these obvious sources the

researcher is reduced to the more difficult task of finding collections in private hands. Advertising in medical and nursing journals often produces good results. Many of these private collections are better cared for than those in institutions.

SECONDARY SOURCES

This brief account of secondary sources covering various aspects of the history of photography and medicine is addressed to two audiences. First, we address those who do not usually exploit photographic material but who work on the modern history of medicine, or the recent social history of Britain and the United States. For these historians, we survey some of the works we have found helpful on the history and interpretation of photography. Second is an audience we hope to acquire: intellectual historians and scholars of the history of art and photography who might be persuaded to become interested in medical photographs. For this audience, we have noted recent historiographic essays on the history of medicine and adjacent disciplines and we have also identified the major general bibliographies. We do not include here specific works in the history of medicine which we have used to interpret photographs in context. Our debt to our colleagues is too vast to discharge by a summary list.

There is a rich literature on the history of photography and many of the best books have excellent bibliographies. A standard general work is Helmut and Alison Gernsheim, *A Concise History of Photography from the Camera Obscura to the Beginning of the Modern Era* (London: Thames and Hudson, 1955). Invaluable because of its attempt to integrate social, technological and aesthetic history is Beaumont Newhall's *The History of Photography from 1839 to the Present Day* (New York: The Museum of Modern Art, 1964). A useful shorter history is Ian Jeffrey, *Photography: A Concise History* (London: Thames and Hudson, 1981). Several monographs have been written about the history of photography in the United States. These include: Robert Taft, *Photography and the American Scene* (New York: Macmillan, 1938; Dover, 1964); Richard Rudisill, *Mirror Image: The Influence of the Daguerreotype on American Society* (Albuquerque: University of New Mexico Press, 1971); and Reese V. Jenkins, *Images and Enterprise: Technology and the American Photographic Industry, 1839-1925* (Baltimore: Johns Hopkins University Press, 1975). Although an exhibition catalogue, a comparable British work is Mark Haworth-Booth, *The Golden Age of British Photography 1839-1900* (New York: Aperture and Victoria and Albert Museum, 1984). Other catalogues of American and British exhibitions, too numerous to mention, contain useful historical information and analysis.

The literature on interpreting photographs is, in the main, based on theories and methods developed by art historians. Much contemporary analysis draws heavily on works of Erwin Panofsky and E. H. Gombrich, especially Panofsky's *Meaning in the Visual Arts* (Garden City, N.Y.: Doubleday, 1955). A useful history and analysis of his concepts of iconography and iconology is Christine Hasenmueller, "Panofsky, Iconography and Semiotics," *Journal of Aesthetics and Art Criticism,* 1978, 36:289-301. Gombrich's influential works include, *Art and Illusion: A Study of the Psychology of Pictorial Representation* (Princeton: Princeton University Press, 1960), *Art, Perception and Reality* (Baltimore: Johns Hopkins University Press, 1972) and, with R. L. Gregory, *Illusion in Nature and Art* (London: Duckworth, 1973).

Works concerned with the production processes in the graphic arts are invaluable for understanding photographs, William Ivins's, *Prints and Visual Communcation* (Cambridge: Harvard University Press, 1953) remains a mine of ideas about what he called "exactly repeatable pictorial statements." Ivins's ideas were revised and extended by Estelle Jussim in *Visual Communication and the Graphic Arts: Photographic Technologies in the Nineteenth Century* (New York and London: R. R. Bowker Company, 1974).

The literature which specifically deals with the nature of photographic representation is large and contentious. A pioneering work is John Szarkowski, *The Photographer's Eye* (Boston: New York Graphic Society, for the Museum of Modern Art, 1966). Szarkowski's five analytical categories have been extraordinarily influential. His category of "time" is, however, aesthetic rather than historical. Szarkowski regards photographs as pictures of "slices of time," which are separate from other events. To Szarkowski, photographs do not tell stories; they only make stories clear.

Many of the scholars whose work has influenced the interpretation of photographs, including Ivins and Gombrich, regard photography as different from other visual arts. Joel Snyder is a penetrating critic of this point of view. In an important article, written with Neil Walsh Allen, "Photography, Vision and Representation," *Critical Inquiry,* Autumn 1975, 2:143-68, Snyder concluded that "even if we are interested in photographs as 'documents' rather than as 'art,' the naive belief that photography lies outside the sphere of other representations can lead to a basic misunderstanding of the 'documentary' questions we ought to ask." Snyder extended this argument in "Picturing Vision," *Critical Inquiry,* Spring 1980, 6:499-526, and in "Benjamin on Reproducibility and Aura: A Reading of 'The Work of Art in the Age of its Technical Reproductibility,'" *Philosophical Forum,* Fall-Winter, 1983-84, 15:130-145. A challenging but, we believe, unconvincing critique of Snyder is Kendall L. Walton, "Transparent Pictures: On the Nature of Photographic Realism," *Critical Inquiry,* December 1984, 11:246-277.

An important work on the historical context of photography is Stephen Bann, *The Clothing of Clio* (Cambridge: University Press, 1984). Bann, while appreciating that photographic reproduction "aroused no absolutely new types of response" (p. 133), nevertheless argues that photography was at "the extreme boundary" of an entirely new form of historical discourse (p. 136). He draws attention to Ranke's "wie es eigentlich gewesen" theory of history and our own "having-been-there" impression of photographs. This work, incidentally, is also extremely illuminating on the relation of illustrations to the historical text.

Both Susan Sontag and Roland Barthes have written controversial essays on interpreting photographs. Sontag's *On Photography* (New York: Farrar, Straus and Giroux, 1977) has been an influential statement about the independence of photography as an art. Sontag was, however, ambiguous in her discussion of the nature of the photographic representation. On the one hand, she asserted that "photographs are as much an interpretation of the world as paintings and drawings are" (pp. 6-7), and, on the other, that "a photograph is not only . . . an interpretation of the real; it is also a trace, something directly stencilled off the real" (p. 154). Barthes, whose general views on interpreting photographs are similar to Sontag's, resolved this ambiguity to his own satisfaction. Ultimately, he argued, photographs record reality. They have a denotative as well as a connotative function. In a book published in English as *Camera Lucida: Reflections on Photography* (New York: Hill and Wang, 1981), he wrote, "It is the fashion nowadays, to seize upon a semantic relativity: no 'reality' . . . nothing but artifice . . . in the photograph, the power of authentication exceeds the power of representation." Barthes, *Mythologies* (London: Jonathon Cape, 1972) is full, however, of penetrating insights into photographic iconography.

Sontag's and Barthes's work has been widely discussed. Sontag was both attacked and defended by the contributors to Jerome Leibling, ed., *Photography: Current Perspectives* (Rochester, New York: Light Impressions Corporation, for the Massachusetts Review, 1978). Bob Rogers criticized "faith in photographic realism" in "Realism and the Photographic Image," *Gazette des Beaux-Arts,* 1981, 98:89-94. A thorough analysis of Sontag's aesthetic theory is Stephanie Ross, "What Photographs Can't Do," *Journal of Aesthetics and Art Criticism,* Fall, 1982, 41:5-17. The most recent essays of Joel Snyder, cited above, seem to us to be the most convincing critique of Barthes and Sontag.

Several critics who have explored the nature of photographic representation have combined art-historical and Marxist concepts. The most notable are John Berger and Alan Sekula. Important statements by Berger include *Ways of Seeing* (London: British Broadcasting Corporation and Penguin Books, 1972 and subsequent editions) and *About Looking* (New York: Pantheon, 1980). His essay "Uses of Photography" in the latter book is a commentary on Sontag. Berger regards photographs as conveying an instant of time abstracted from a narrative process. This narrative we as spectators construct for ourselves, with more or less help from other sources. With the photographer Jean Mohr, Berger also produced *Another Way of Telling* (London: Writers and Readers, 1982), in which he explores the "truth" of the photograph. Sekula's essays include, "On the Invention of Photographic Meaning," in Victor Burgin, ed., *Thinking Photography* (London: The Macmillan Press, 1982) and "The Traffic in Photographs," *Art Journal,* Spring 1981, 41:15-25. Both Berger and Sekula explicitly relate the history of photography to the history of capitalism. For Berger, photography's "ethical reputation for truth" derives from its conscious use to assist in "the secularization of the capitalist world during the nineteenth century" (*About Looking,* p. 54), Sekula contends that "photography is haunted by two chattering ghosts: that of bourgeois science and that of bourgeois art" ("The Traffic," p. 15). In a similar vein, see Robert M. Levine, "Semiotics for the Historian: Photographers as Cultural Messengers," *Reviews in American History,* 1985, 13:375-380. A more specific historical study, which employs a Foucauldian model to explore the use of the photograph in the policing of modern society is John Tagg, "Power and Photography," *Screen,* 1980, 81, 36, 37:17-55, 17-27. An extension of Tagg's argument to medicine is found in Roberta McGrath, "Medical Police," *Ten. 8,* 1984, 14:13-18. Although not dealing with the photograph alone, a sociological approach to the replication of social relations in visual images can be found in Irving Goffman, *Gender Advertisements* (London: Macmillan, 1979). For an illuminating account of editorial decisions in photojournalism, see Harold Evans, *Pictures on a Page* (London: Heinemann, 1978).

A few scholars have tried to reassert the "truthfulness" of photographs. Stanley Cavell argues that a photograph "is not a likeness; it is not exactly a replica or a relic or a shadow, or an apparition either" in *The World Viewed: Reflections on the Ontology of Film* (Cambridge: Harvard University Press, 1979), p. 18. Roger Scruton has argued that photographs are a "presentation" rather than "representation" in "Photography and Representation," *Critical Inquiry,* Spring 1981, 7:577-603.

A number of historians have written about the problems and opportunities of interpreting photographs as historical sources. One of the first to do so was Judith M. Gutman in *Lewis W. Hine and the American Social Conscience* (New York: Walker and Company, 1967) and *Lewis W. Hine: Two Perspectives* (New York: Grossman, 1974). In the introduction to *Wisconsin Death Trip* (New York: Pantheon, 1973), Michael Lesy argued that photographs themselves could be used to construct a historical narrative. Lesy continued to explore the historiographic problems of using photographs in *Real Life* (New York: Pantheon, 1976) in a short essay "'Mere' Snapshots, Considered" in the *New York Times,* January 16, 1978, and in the introduction to *Bearing Witness: A Photographic*

Chronicle of American Life (New York: Pantheon, 1982). Other historians have urged that the techniques of art history and photographic criticism be adapted for the study of historical photographs. The earliest paper we have found is Marsha Peters and Bernard Mergen, "Doing the Rest': The Uses of Photographs in American Studies," *American Quarterly,* Summer 1977, 29:280-303. Daniel M. Fox and James Terry suggested a method for iconographic analysis of photographs in "Photography and the Self Image of American Physicians, 1880-1920," *Bulletin of the History of Medicine,* Spring 1978, 52:435-57. This method, adopted mainly from Gombrich and Szarkowski, has been radically changed as a result of the writing of this book. A major essay, with implications beyond the study of photographs, is Neil Harris, "Iconography and Intellectual History: The Half-Tone Effect," in John Higham and Paul K. Conkin, eds., *New Directions in American Intellectual History* (Baltimore and London: The Johns Hopkins University Press, 1979), pp. 196-211. A useful paper is Richard Rudisill, "On Reading Photographs," *Journal of American Culture,* Fall 1982, 5:1-14. A brief article which argues that photographs can only supplement written sources is Madelyn Moeller, "Photography and History: Using Photographs in Interpreting our Cultural Past," *Journal of American Culture,* Spring 1983, 6:3-17. A good close reading of selected photographs is Jonathan Bayer, *Reading Photographs: Understanding the Aesthetics of Photography* (New York: Pantheon Books, 1977) as is Julia Hirsch, *Family Photographs: Content, Meaning and Effect* (New York: Oxford University Press, 1981). Photographers, of course, can also make the reader aware of the conventions being employed. See Richard Avedon, *In the American West* (London: Thames and Hudson, 1985). The reader with an 'image' of the American West will be surprised by Avedon's photographs.

A few scholars of art and photography have also addressed the question of how to analyze historical photographs. A notable paper is James C. A. Kaufmann, "Photographs and History," first published in *Exposure,* Summer 1978, but more accessible in T. F. Barrow et al., *Reading into Photography: Selected Essays, 1959-1980* (Albuquerque: University of New Mexico Press, 1982), pp. 193-99. A critique of the imposition of categories from art history on nineteenth century photographs which were taken for documentary purposes is Rosalind Krauss, "Photography's Discursive Spaces: Landscape/View," *Art Journal,* Winter 1982:311-19.

The study of photographs as historical sources, it seems to us, could benefit from the work of sociologists of knowledge. Some of the most intriguing, if most contentious, work on the sociology of knowledge concerns itself with the hard case, science itself. Since photographs are so frequently regarded as representing the world with the same sort of truthfulness as scientific statements this work seems eminently appropriate if it can be applied. Theoretical statements of how social interests are the basis of scientific theories are Barry Barnes, *Scientific Knowledge* and *Sociological theory* (Lond: Routledge, Kegan Paul, 1974) and *Interests and the Growth of Knowledge* (London: Routledge, Kegan Paul, 1977). A valuable treatment of conventions is to be found in David Bloor, *Knowledge and Social Imagery* (London: Routledge, Kegan Paul, 1976). Both of these authors adhere to a thoroughly socially constructivist account of scientific knowledge. Unfortunately, there is not yet any general text dealing with the social construction of scientific imagery, but see the essays in 'Les 'vues' De L'Esprit', *Culture Technique*, 1985, 14. However, a few historians of science have begun to make detailed case studies of particular sorts of illustration, for example, M. J. S. Rudwick, "A Visual Language for Geology" in *History of Science*, 1976, 14: 149-95; and Steven Shapin, "The Politics of Observation, Cerebral Anatomy and Social Interests in the Edinburgh Phrenology Dispute" in R. Wallis, ed., *On the Margins of Science* (Sociological Review Monographs, 1978). Conversely, there is a specific study by an art historian which has attempted to relate seventeenth-century scientific accounts of the world to a new way of seeing and representing, Svetlana Alpers, *The Art of Describing. Dutch Art in the Seventeenth Century* (London: John Murray, 1983). This work, however, has been strongly criticised, see E. De Jongh, *Simiolus, Netherlands Quarterly for the History of Art*, 1984, *14*: 51-59.

Historians have used photographs in different ways. The most common use has been to illustrate a narrative based almost entirely on written sources. Most of the scholars for whom photographs are merely supplemental assume that they "capture moments of unposed reality," as Colin Ford and Brian Harrison wrote in *A Hundred Years Ago: Britain in the 1880s in Words and Photographs* (Cambridge: Harvard University Press, 1983), p. 12. For a typical statement of this widely used approach, and which seems to us the antithesis of ours, see Gordon Winter, *A Cockney Camera* (Harmondsworth, Penguin, 1975). In his introduction Winter writes:

Any attempt at social history based on the evidence in old photographs tends to write itself. It is impossible to set out with preconceived ideas of what life was like in the Victorian-Edwardian era, and then produce a collection of photographs to illustrate those ideas; all one can do is to seek out the widest possible range of early photographs, choose the ones that seem interesting and relevant, and then present them in an order that will let them tell their own story.

Michael Lesy, similarly, has no narrative prose at all in his most recent book. Lesy has not, however, always been confident that a series of photographs alone can tell an adequate story about a series of events. In

Real Life, for example, he complained that photographs were the "least convincing" of the sources he used. He added, however, that "the text is intended to elaborate not illustrate the photographs" (vii).

A few scholars have combined photographs with text, but ultimately they remain illustrations. These include Alan Thomas's innovative *Time in a Frame: Photography and the Nineteenth Century Mind* (New York: Schocken Books, 1977), see also Arthur Marwick, *Britain in our Century: Images and Controversies* (New York: Thames and Hudson, 1984). Perhaps the most innovative use of photographs and prose in a historical account is David Galloway, *A Family Album* (New York: Harcourt Brace Jovanovich, 1978). Galloway's book, part novel part monograph, is about family life in the American South in this century. He tells his story by establishing the context of six photographs and then analyzing each of them. John Berger and Jean Mohr's, *A Fortunate Man* (London: Writers and Readers, 1967) is an account of modern British rural general practice. Two recent similar books are Peter Hales, *Silver Cities: The Photography of American Urbanization, 1839-1915* (Philadelphia: Temple University Press, 1984) and David E. Nye, *Image Worlds: Identities at General Electric* (Cambridge: MIT Press, 1985). See also Donald E. English, *Political Uses of Photography in the Third French Republic, 1881-1914* (Ann Arbor: University of Michigan Research Press, 1984) and M. Weaver, *The Photographic Art: Pictorial Traditions in Britain and America* (New York: Harper Row, 1986).

Historians of medicine have long been interested in the participation of doctors in inventing and refining photographic technology and using it to record clinical events. The first effort to summarize what was known about the history of photography and medicine appears to have been George Rosen, ed., "Medicine and Early Photography," *Ciba Symposia*, August-September 1942, 4:1330-59. This pamphlet contained articles by Beaumont Newhall, "A Brief History of Photographic Techniques," George Rosen, "Early Medical Photography," and H. Gurtner, "Etienne Jules Marey and Edward Muybridge, Pioneers in Motion Analysis." Fox and Terry in "Photography and the Self Image of American Physicians, 1880-1920," summarized the primary and secondary literature on doctors and photography, pp. 440-42. Sander Gilman has published two studies of early photography of the insane: *The Face of Madness: Hugh W. Diamond and the Origin of Psychiatric Photography* (New York: Brunner-Mazel, 1976); and a chapter, "Photography and Madness," in his *Seeing the Insane* (New York: John Wiley and Sons, 1982). For a study of Charcot and photography in French medicine see Georges Didi-Huberman, *Invention de l'Hysterie. Charcot et l'Iconographie Photographique de la Salpetriere* (Paris: Editions Macula, 1982). Stanley Burns has written a detailed monograph, "Early Medical Photography in America," *New York State Medical Journal*, 1979, 79:788-95, and six subsequent issues. These papers are collected in Stanley Burns, *Early Medical Photography in America* (New York: The Burns Archive, 1983). There is no comparable study of early medical photography in Britain. See, however, the interesting work by Pam Schweitzer, ed., *Can We Afford the Doctor?* (London: Age Exchange, 1985) which combines medical photographs with recollections by Londoners of medical care over the last seventy years. A study which pays attention to British photographic portraits of doctors is Gertrude M. Prescott, "A Question of Image: British Portrait Publications, 1856-1896" (Ph.D. dissertation, University of Texas at Austin, 1985). Stanley Joel Reiser, *Medicine and the Reign of Technology* (New York: Cambridge University Press, 1978), addresses doctors' interest in photography in the context of the growing use of technology in medicine in the nineteenth century.

Readers who work with photographs but who do not work in the history of medicine may want to consult historiographic essays and bibliographies. A useful introduction to the field is Gert Brieger, "History of Medicine," in Paul T. Durbin, ed., *A Guide to the Culture of Science, Technology and Medicine* (New York: Free Press, 1980), which should be read in conjunction with the essays in the same volume by Arnold Thackray, "History of Science," and Carroll W. Pursell, Jr., "History of Technology." A guide to historiography and pertinent literature is Pietro Corsi and Paul Weindling, eds., *Information Sources in the History of Science and Medicine* (London: Butterworth Scientific, 1983). There are several indispensable bibliographies: Wellcome Institute for the History of Medicine and Related Sciences, *Subject Catalogue of the History of Medicine and Related Sciences* (Munich: Kraus International Publications, 1980) supplemented by *Current Work in the History of Medicine,* a quarterly bibliography; United States Department of Health and Human Services, National Library of Medicine, *Bibliography of the History of Medicine* (Washington, D.C.: United States Government Office, 1965-   ); and Genevieve Miller, *Bibliography of the History of Medicine of the United States and Canada, 1939-60* (Baltimore: Johns Hopkins University Press, 1964).

NOTES

CHAPTER I

1. Raymond Williams, *Culture* (London: Fontana Paperbacks, 1981), p. 13.
2. Examples of this scholarship are presented below in Chapter VI.
3. The quotation is from William Ivins, *Prints and Visual Communication.* (Cambridge, Mass.: Harvard University Press, 1953) p. 94.
4. Zola is quoted in Beaumont Newhall, *The History of Photography* (New York: Museum of Modern Art, 1964), p. 94.
5. *Medical Times and Gazette,* 1866, 1:319.
6. Richard Wolfe, Countway Library, Harvard Medical School, personal communication.
7. This is suggested by an image which appears in W. R. Merrington, *University College Hospital and its Medical School: A History* (London: Heinemann, 1976). Figure 23 is entitled "Dr. Herbert Spencer's last caesarean section 1925." In it the surgeon stands in a stained gown in front of, presumably, colleagues and students. This is a photograph which celebrates Dr. Herbert Spencer, servant of the hospital, not operative obstetrics.

CHAPTER II

1. On the role of recording in nineteenth century culture, see Carlo Ginzberg, "Morelli, Freud and Sherlock Holmes: Clues and the Scientific Method," *History Workshop,* 1980, 9:5-36.
2. *The Lancet,* 1859, 1:89.
3. See for example *British Medical Journal,* 1864, 1:547; 1876, 1:301; 1879, 2:783; 1888, 1:1019; 1891, 1:363.
4. William Henry Fox Talbot called the earliest form of his paper photographs exhibited in January 1839 "photogenic drawing." Cited in Mark Haworth-Booth, ed., *The Golden Age of British Photography* (London: Aperture, 1984), p. 30.
5. In 1865 the annual report of the London Photographic Society recorded "the number of photographers of eminence among the ranks of the medical profession." *The Lancet,* 1865, 1:218. Early photographic journals contained numerous articles by physicians. For a list of articles in various languages, see Daniel M. Fox and James S. Terry, "Photography and the Self-Image of American Physicians," *Bulletin of the History of Medicine,* Spring 1978, 52:441.

6. On Keith, see C. S. Minto, *Thomas Keith 1827-1895: Surgeon and Photographer* (Edinburgh: City Libraries, 1966). See also A. D. Morrison-Low, "Dr. John and Robert Adamson: An Early Partnership in Scottish Photography," *The Photographic Collector*, 1983, *4*:134-147. On Draper, see Stanley Burns, *Early Medical Photography in America* (New York: The Burns Archive, 1983).

7. *British Medical Journal*, 1867, *2*:464. On American *carte-de-visite*, see Burns, *Early Medical Photography in America*.

8. *British Medical Journal, 1873, 1*:718.

9. Medical men appeared both in the many volumes devoted to eminent men as well in those solely about medical figures. For a study and a bibliography of this literature, see Gertrude M. Prescott, "A Question of Image: British Portrait Publications 1856-1896" (Ph.D Thesis, University of Texas at Austin, 1985). The publication of such pictures provoked accusations of advertising. See for example the case of the dismissal of John Gay from the Royal Free Hospital. Gay's portrait and biographical memoir had appeared in the *Medical Circular* as an engraving from a photograph. See *The Lancet* 1854, *1*:86; *Medical Times and Gazette,* 1854, *1*:16. On the sensitivity of the medical profession to such issues at this time see M. Jeanne Peterson, *The Medical Profession in Mid-Victorian London* (Berkeley: University of California Press, 1978).

10. *British Medical Journal*, 1864, *2*:15.

11. See *British Medical Journal*, 1882 *1*:469; and Alex Sakula, "The Baroness Burdett-Coutts' Garden Party: The International Medical Congress London 1881," *Medical History*, 1982, *26*:183-90.

12. See for example *British Medical Journal*, 1863 *1*:97; *The Lancet,* 1869, *1*:145-46. In America a journal, *Photographic Review of Medicine and Surgery* was started in 1870, and was published monthly for two years.

13. For instance, Robert Carswell, *Pathological Anatomy. Illustrations of the Elementary Forms of Disease* (London: Longman, 1838).

14. *British Medical Journal*, 1886 *1*:162.

15. Lionel S. Beale, *How to Work with the Microscope* (London: Harrison, 4th ed., 1868), p. 33. The camera which supposedly was faithful in its representation of nature, was useless in adjudicating in disputes about the nature of protoplasm. See Gerald L. Geison, "The Protoplasmic Theory of Life and the Vitalist—Mechanist debate," *Isis,* 1969, *60*:273-91. Similarly, the surgeon, Lennox Browne, was one of the first to photograph the larynx, but his obituary recorded "his most permanently valuable contributions to science are to be found in his coloured drawings of diseased conditions," *British Medical Journal*, 1902, *2*:1566. The first tipped-in photograph to appear in the *British Medical Journal* was of a larynx taken by Browne, *British Medical Journal*, 1883, *2*:811.

16. On geology see M. J. S. Rudwick, "A Visual Language for Geology," *History of Science*, 1976, *14*:149-95; and idem., *The Great Devonian Controversy* (Chicago: University of Chicago Press, 1985).

17. Cesare Lombroso, an Italian criminologist whose works were extensively used in America, employed photographs as evidence that there was a typology of depraved individuals. See, for example, C. Lombroso, *Criminal Man* (New York: G. P. Putnam's Sons, 1911); and James Bennett, *Oral History and Delinquency: The Rhetoric of Criminology* (Chicago: University of Chicago Press, 1981), p. 120.

18. But not apparently in Europe, see Burns, *Early Medical Photography* p. 1258.

19. Cited in Sander L. Gilman, *The Face of Madness: Hugh W. Diamond and the Origins of Psychiatric Photography* (New York: Brunner/Mazel, 1976), p. 7.

20. John Conolly, "The Physiognomy of Insanity," *Medical Times and Gazette*, 1858, *1*:3.

21. Sander L. Gilman, *Seeing the Insane* (New York: John Wiley and Sons, 1982). The most famous use of photographs to represent mental states was J. M. Charcot's photographs of hysterics. See the volume by Didi-Huberman cited in Chapter VI.

22. *The Lancet*, 1858, *2*:68. For examples, see Burns, *Early Medical Photography*.

23. See Leslie Fiedler, *Freaks: Myths and Images of the Secret Self* (London: Penguin Books, 1981); Martin Howard, *Victorian Grotesque* (London: Jupiter Books, 1977).

24. "A Remarkable Case of Double Monstrosity in an Adult," *Lancet*, 1865, *2*:124-25. For the response see *British Medical Journal*, 1865, *2*:185. Photographs of this man, Jean Battista dos Santos, are at the Royal Society of Medicine and the Leeds Medical School.

25. *British Medical Journal*, 1865, *2*:165.

26. Martin L. Scott, "Technology the Enabler," *Image*, 1981, 24:4-9. In conversation Scott agrees that the "ability to take close-ups preceded the convention of doing so."

CHAPTER III

1. This paragraph generalizes about a great many photographs. Hospital photographs were taken from the 1850s in the United States and from a somewhat later date in Britain. We emphasize the period after 1880, when hospital imagery dominated medical photography. Postcards at this time were photographs, not prints made by the half-tone process.

2. For pictures of a Poor Law Infirmary see, for example, Janet Gooch, *A History of Brighton General Hospital* (London: Phillimore, 1980).

3. There is not much literature on the hospital ward in Victorian England. Iron beds, flowers, carpets, spare armchairs, and polished wooden floors all figure in the Nightingale model. See Florence Nightingale, *Notes on Hospitals* (London: Longman, 3d ed. 1863); idem., *Notes on Nursing: What It Is and What It Is Not* (London: Harrison, [1860]). On the hospital as the site of moral management rather than one of therapeutic intervention, see Charles Rosenberg, "Florence Nightingale on Contagion; The Hospital as Moral Universe," in Charles Rosenberg, ed., *Healing and History* (New York: Science History Publications, 1979), pp. 116-36. For the relative lack of power of the medical profession in the British hospitals of this period, see M. Jeanne Peterson, *The Medical Profession in Mid-Victorian London* (Berkeley: University of California Press 1978). For ward design, see John D. Thompson and Grace Goldin, *The Hospital: A Social and Architectural History* (New Haven: Yale University Press, 1975). That hospitals were thought of as domestic institutions is suggested by the fact that they were often known as "the house." Consider also the use of the terms "workhouse," "poorhouse," "asylum," "cottage hospital."

4. Private accommodation was rare in British voluntary hospitals. Patients paid 3 pounds 3 shillings per week for the partitioned cubicles of Bright ward. See H. C. Cameron, *Mr. Guy's Hospital* (London: Longmans, 1954).

5. On American domestic work, see Ruth Schwartz Cowan, *More Work for Mother* (New York: Basic Books, 1983); on industrial photographs, David E. Nye, *Image Worlds: Corporate Identities at General Electric* (Cambridge: MIT Press, 1985).

6. Florence Nightingale certainly perceived nursing as analogous to the best domestic service. The Victorian country house was subdivided into a great number of small specialized rooms with numerous classes of servants. Service in a great house was often an occupation of which to be proud. See Mark Girouard, *Life in the English Country House* (New Haven: Yale University Press, 1978); idem., *The Victorian Country House* (Oxford: Clarendon Press, 1971). On the hierarchical structure of an English hospital, see Lindsay Granshaw, *St. Mark's Hospital: A Social History of a Specialist Hospital* (London: Kings Fund Historical Series, Number 2, 1985), chap. 8. Many English hospital governors, of course, would themselves have had large households; but so would their American counterparts, which makes baffling the difference in how hospital work was represented in photographs.

7. For a good example of the sanatorium ideology of the outdoor life, see the text and pictures in J. R. Bignall, *Frimley: The Biography of a Sanatorium* (London: National Heart and Chest Hospitals, 1979). The hospital issued a composite postcard, showing "How consumptives built a reservoir" (p. 59).

8. Orkney's original negatives remain at Montrose. None of his work has been published, although it is worthy of it. The dating of many of these pictures is problematic. Some undoubtedly date from after the First World War. However, they are unique as hospital pictures whether for the 1920s or the Edwardian era. There is a short account of the asylum in A. S. Presly, *A Sunnyside Chronicle: A History of Sunnyside Royal Hospital, Produced for its Bi-Centenary* ([1981]). There are no Orkney pictures in this volume.

9. The contrast here is with the years after the First World War when British nurses were photographed in classrooms. They may have been photographed in this way before the war but, if so, such pictures are rare. There is a photograph of nurses learning the practical skill of bandaging in S. A. Tooley, *History of Nursing in the British Empire* (London: S. H. Bonsfield, 1906), facing p. 164.

10. On the British hospital physician as a man of letters, see Christopher Lawrence, "Incommunicable Knowledge: Science Technology and the Clinical Art in Britain, 1850-1914," *Journal of Contemporary History*, 1985, *20*:503-20. Steven Paget nicely described the separation of clinic and genteel study in Victor Horsley's house in Cavendish Square.

His consulting-room was the front room on the ground floor; it looked on the Square, which is pleasant enough to look at, when the leaves are on the trees; it was comfortable, cheerful, white-walled, and neither too large nor too small. Among his belongings in it were models in yellow marble of temple-columns in the Roman Forum, and a very beautiful drawing of San Miniato in Florence, by Gerald Horsley; and, on the mantlepiece, bronzes from Rome, and some treasured little casts of a monkey's brain. Opening into the consulting room, there was a well fitted dark-room, for the examination of the eye, ear, and throat.

Sir Victor Horsley (London: Constable, 1919) p. 142.

11. In November 1915, Lord Derby, Director-General of Recruiting sent a letter to second and third year medical students advising them that it was their duty to

join His Majesty's Forces. The Dean of St. Bartholomew's urged upon Derby the importance of maintaining a continuous supply of medical men, *British Medical Journal*, 1915, *2*:686.

12. Perhaps the most popular idealization was William Small's "The Good Samaritan" (Leicester Art Gallery) of which numerous engravings were produced. The picture showed a doctor at the roadside, attending a gypsy family in a tent. One of the few photographs of a man we presume to be a general practitioner shows him as an incidental element in a photograph of a Guy's nurse attending a gypsy maternity case in a tent. See *The Hospital*, 1906, *39*:320. On the ideal of the general practitioner, see Irvine Loudon, "The Concept of the Family Doctor," *Bulletin of the History of Medicine*, 1984, *58*:347-62.

13. By the early twentieth century, motor manufacturers were modifying cars for the medical profession, see for example the photograph "Specially Adapted for Doctors: A New 16-HP Humber Car with a Two-Seated Coupé Body," in *The Illustrated London News*, May 14, 1910, p. 746. On the change brought by the automobile in American medicine, see Paul Starr, *The Social Transformation of American Medicine* (New York: Basic Books, 1982), pp. 69-71.

14. D'Arcy Power and W. E. Le Fanu, *Lives of the Fellows of the Royal College of Surgeons of England 1930-1951* (London: RCS, 1953), p. 567.

15. For change in surgical clothing, see James M. Edmonson, *Surgical Garb 1870-1920* (Cleveland: Cleveland Health Sciences Library, 1982).

16. Frederic S. Dennis, "The History and Development of Surgery during the Past Century," *American Medicine*, 1905, *9*:139-46. Dennis was professor of clinical surgery at Cornell University.

17. On the exhibition of the "Gross Clinic," see David Sellin, *The First Pose* (New York: W. W. Norton and Company, 1976), p. 15; and Elizabeth Johns, *Thomas Eakins: The Heroism of Modern Life* (Princeton: Princeton University Press, 1983), pp. 75-76.

18. This and the following few pictures are subsidiary to our main theme. They are not part of a distinct *medical* imagery. Their uses may have lain in other spheres, the celebration of the engineering profession or local government for instance. But the imagery of hygiene as a civic ideal was complemented by pictures of, say, nurses delousing in public buildings.

19. The photographic records of the Eugenics Society are in the Wellcome Institute Library. See also for instance, Lieutenant-Colonel Douglas, "The Degenerates and the Modes of their Elimination," *Physician and Surgeon*. 1900, *1*:481-89. This piece was liberally illustrated with half-tones, depicting such figures as "A degenerate fit for anything from pitch-and-toss to manslaughter."

20. Boer war photography does not seem to have produced a coherent medical image. Photographs for public display, as a recent writer on the subject put it, "seem embalmed in nineteenth century heroic rhetoric." The war did, however, produce a large number of "snapshots" taken by private soldiers with the first easily portable cameras with roll-film. See Emanoel Lee, *To the Bitter End. A Photographic History of the Boer War, 1899-1902* (New York: Viking, 1985), p. 4.

21. On cardiology, see Christopher Lawrence "Moderns and ancients: The 'New Cardiology' in Britain 1880-1930," and Joel D. Howell, "'Soldiers Heart': The Redefinition of Heart Disease and Speciality Formation in Early Twentieth Century Great Britain," in W. F. Bynum, Christopher Lawrence, and V. Nutton, eds., *The Emergence of Modern Cardiology* (London: Medical History Supplement

Number 5, 1985). On psychiatry, see Martin Stone, "Shell Shock and the Psychologists," in W. F. Bynum, Roy Porter, and Michael Shepherd, eds., *The Anatomy of Madness: Essays in the History of Psychiatry*, vol. 2, *Institutions and Society* (London: Tavistock, 1985).

CHAPTER IV

1. On photographs of work in Britain, see Arts Council of Great Britain, *The British Worker: Photographs of Working Life, 1839-1939* (London: Arts Council 1981); for America, see Judith Mara Gutman, *Lewis W. Hine and the American Social Conscience* (New York: Walker, 1967).

2. On January 3rd, 1925, *The Illustrated London News* ran a three-page article on the bicentenary of Guy's hospital. There were twelve photographs, among them: the waiting room for "the new massage and electrical department," "electrical whirlpool baths," "the X-ray lamp in the deep X-ray department," "ultraviolet rays" and the deep X-ray department control room.

3. Work on radioactivity following the discoveries of the Curies and the atomic studies of Niels Bohr and Ernest Rutherford was frequently presented to the public during these years. Radium therapy, Niels Finsen's artificial light therapy, short wave diathermy, and innumerable variants of these physical therapies pervade the text books and photographs of the period. See Margaret Rowbottom and Charles Susskind, *Electricity and Medicine: A History of Their Interaction* (San Francisco: San Francisco Press, 1984). The prestige accorded to these therapies made them great favorites of unqualified practitioners. See, for example, the satire in A. J. Cronin's, *The Citadel*, first published in 1937.

4. Example of nurses with sexual identity in popular culture are presented in Philip A. Kalisch and Beatrice J. Kalisch, *The Advance of American Nursing* (Boston: Little Brown, 1978).

5. For Steichen's views, see Edward Steichen, *A Life in Photography* (New York: Doubleday and Company, 1963). In addition to his optimism about science and the human condition, Steichen was also an accomplished advertising photographer (chapter 9), who encouraged viewers to see dramatic stories in his pictures.

6. Just as before the war, general practitioners were rarely photographed. Irvine Loudon, who was a general practitioner and is now a practising historian working on the history of general practice, confirms our view that photographs of British doctors in their surgeries are virtually nonexistent. Dick Maurice, a former G.P. in Wiltshire where his family has had a practice in Marlborough since 1792, could find no photographs of himself or his forebears at work. Significantly his article, "Six Generations in Wiltshire," *British Medical Journal*, 1982, 1:284-86, included a photograph of his grandfather in 1905 standing beside his carriage outside the surgery. Compare the convention used in Fig. 3.62.

7. *Picture Post*, December 2, 1939, p. 26.

8. See the photographs reproduced in John D. Stoeckle and George Abbott White, *Plain Pictures of Plain Doctoring* (Cambridge: MIT Press, 1985). These are pictures from the Farm Security Administration of the New Deal. The medical pictures form a small part of the whole collection. The authors concluded that the object of the photographs was both to condemn rural poverty and celebrate New

Deal intervention. In most respects the photographs conform to our analysis. They are mainly pictures of private consultations, usually alone or in the presence of the family. The invasion was permissible since they were publicly funded medical services. A newspaper reporter, however, documented that the families of the subjects of Walker Evans's most famous FSA photographs continued to believe they were exploited by the photographers (Howell Raines, "Let Us Now Revisit Famous Folk", *The New York Times Magazine*, May 25, 1980, pp. 31-40; 42; 46.). The poor did not necessarily perceive their lives in the way that photographers did.

9. "Geriatrics: Welfare Hospital Specialized in Oldsters' Chronic Diseases," *Life*, October 7, 1940, 9:45-48.

10. This, in its turn, became a cliché. See the dramatic picture of nurses at an operation, "Women in White" by the Chicago surgeon Max Thorek in Victor Robinson, *White Caps: The Story of Nursing* (Philadelphia: J. B. Lippincott, 1946), plates unnumbered.

CHAPTER V

1. David Armstrong, *The Political Anatomy of the Body* (Cambridge: Cambridge University Press, 1983), deals creatively with the literature of social medicine.

2. *Picture Post*, January 7, 1939, pp. 18-22. Many of the pictures in this chapter from *Picture Post* were similar to those in *Life* and other magazines. We publish here a preponderence of photographs from *Picture Post* for the simple reason that reproduction rights for *Life* photographs are prohibitively expensive.

3. "U.S. Science Wars Against an Unknown Enemy: Cancer," *Life*, March 1, 1937, 1: pp. llff.

4. John Keegan, *The Face of Battle* (London: Penguin 1976); Christopher Phillips, *Steichen at War* (New York: Harry W. Abrams, Inc., 1981).

5. Stuart Hall, "The Social Eye of *Picture Post*" in *Working Papers in Cultural Studies (2)* (Birmingham: Centre for Contemporary Cultural Studies at the University of Birmingham, Spring 1972). This excellent study which explores *Picture Post*'s radical elements misses the traditional stereotyping of the medical photographs. See also his "The Determinations of News Photographs" in *Working Papers in Cultural Studies (3)* (Birmingham: Centre for Contemporary Cultural Studies at the University of Birmingham, Autumn 1972). *Life* depicted the British home front in the same way as *Picture Post* did, and very differently from the way it depicted the contemporary United States; see, for example, *Life*, January 13, 1941: 22-23, 74.

6. See for instance the double page spread about the opening of the National Institute for Medical Research at Mill Hill London in *The Illustrated London News*, May 6, 1950, pp. 690-91. The theme of high-powered medical research was dealt with through the lives of the research workers and their daily tasks.

7. "Snake Pit" was the title of a ·1948 American film, directed by Anatole Litvak. *Picture Post* published stills from it, May 21, 1949: 23-25.

8. Fashion and sexuality were not necessarily conjoined in photographs. In 1948, *The Illustrated News* dealt with nurses' fashion, but used none of the conventional sexual elements, October 2, p. 384.

9. For a suggestive instance of how perceptions of nurses relate to photographs, see Lucy Ridgley Seymer, *A General History of Nursing* (London: Faber and Faber, 1932). The seond edition of this book, published in 1949, was changed to include an intimate close-up of a nurse spoon-feeding an infant, Fig. 30.

10. There is a remarkably similar picture in the Greater London Photograph Library, 80/7407.

11. "The Birth of a Baby Aims to Reduce Maternal and Infant Mortality," *Life,* April 11, 1938, 4:33-36.

12. This interesting picture may have been read in several ways by contemporaries. The familiar conventions would, presumably, have made the use of British infant welfare practices in Sicily seem entirely legitimate.

13. In Britain an immensely popular television series of the 1960 s "Dr. Finlay's Casebook," based on the novels of A. J. Cronin presented country practice as the ideal medical career. Compare also Cronin's juxtaposition of city and country in his novel, *The Citadel,* first published in 1937.

14. This interpretation is drawn from the text accompanying the photographs. The doctor is described as a man who must "stretch his self-reliance and responsibility to the utmost degree," be "always ready" and "brave icy roads." The doctor is the man who "knows the people and understands their work," from Stephen Hadfield, *Country Doctor* (London: Common Ground, 1950.)

15. John Berger and Jean Mohr, *A Fortunate Man: The Story of a Country Doctor* (London: Allen Lane, 1967).

16. John Berger and Jean Mohr, "The Ambiguity of the Photograph," *Another Way of Telling* (New York: Pantheon, 1982), pp. 85-100.

INDEX

About the Authors

DANIEL M. FOX is Professor of Humanities in Medicine at the State University of New York at Stony Brook. His books include *Engines of Culture: Philanthropy and Art Museums, The Discovery of Abundance: Simon N. Patten and the Transformation of Social Theory* and *Health Policies, Health Politics: The British and American Experience, 1911-65*. He has published many articles on the history of medicine, social policy, and the analysis of photographs.

CHRISTOPHER LAWRENCE is Senior Lecturer in the History of Medicine at the Wellcome Institute for the History of Medicine in London. He is the coauthor of *No Laughing Matter: Historical Aspects of Anesthesia*, and is currently at work on a book about medicine and the Scottish enlightenment. He has also published numerous articles on the history of medicine of the last three centuries, and on medicine's relation to science and technology.